Process Improvement in Heart Failure

Editors

CLYDE W. YANCY
R. KANNAN MUTHARASAN

HEART FAILURE CLINICS

www.heartfailure.theclinics.com

Consulting Editor
EDUARDO BOSSONE

Founding Editor
JAGAT NARULA

October 2020 • Volume 16 • Number 4

ELSEVIER

1600 John F. Kennedy Boulevard • Suite 1800 • Philadelphia, Pennsylvania, 19103-2899

http://www.theclinics.com

HEART FAILURE CLINICS Volume 16, Number 4
October 2020 ISSN 1551-7136, ISBN-13: 978-0-323-75552-8

Editor: Joanna Collett
Developmental Editor: Laura Fisher

Heart Failure Clinics (ISSN 1551-7136) is published quarterly by Elsevier Inc., 360 Park Avenue South, New York, NY 10010-1710. Months of publication are January, April, July, and October. Business and editorial offices: 1600 John F. Kennedy Boulevard, Suite 1800, Philadelphia, PA 19103-2899. Periodicals postage paid at New York, NY, and additional mailing offices. Subscription prices are USD 269.00 per year for US individuals, USD 534.00 per year for US institutions, USD 100.00 per year for US students and residents, USD 300.00 per year for Canadian individuals, USD 618.00 per year for Canadian institutions, USD 315.00 per year for international individuals, USD 618.00 per year for international institutions, and USD 100.00 per year for Canadian and foreign students/residents. To receive student and resident rate, orders must be accompanied by name of affiliated institution, date of term, and the *signature* of program/residency coordinator on institution letterhead. Orders will be billed at individual rate until proof of status is received. Foreign air speed delivery is included in all *Clinics* subscription prices. All prices are subject to change without notice. **POSTMASTER:** Send address changes to *Heart Failure Clinics*, Elsevier Health Sciences Division, Subscription Customer Service, 3251 Riverport Lane, Maryland Heights, MO 63043. **Customer Service: 1-800-654-2452 (US and Canada). From outside of the US and Canada, call 314-447-8871. Fax: 314-447-8029. For print support, E-mail: JournalsCustomerService-usa@elsevier.com. For online support, E-mail: JournalsOnlineSupport-usa@elsevier.com.**

Reprints. For copies of 100 or more of articles in this publication, please contact the Commercial Reprints Department, Elsevier Inc., 360 Park Avenue South, New York, NY 10010-1710. Tel.: 212-633-3874; Fax: 212-633-3820; E-mail: reprints@elsevier.com.

Heart Failure Clinics is covered in *MEDLINE/PubMed (Index Medicus)*.

Contributors

CONSULTING EDITOR

EDUARDO BOSSONE, MD, PhD, FCCP, FESC, FACC
Division of Cardiology, AORN Antonio
Cardarelli Hospital, Naples, Italy

EDITORS

CLYDE W. YANCY, MD, MSc, MACC, FAHA, MACP, FHFSA
Vice Dean, Diversity and Inclusion, Magerstadt
Professor of Medicine, Professor of Medical
Social Sciences, Chief, Division of Cardiology,
Northwestern University Feinberg School of
Medicine, Chicago, Illinois, USA

R. KANNAN MUTHARASAN, MD, FACC
Associate Professor of Medicine, Division of
Cardiology, Department of Medicine,
Northwestern University Feinberg School of
Medicine, Chicago, Illinois, USA

AUTHORS

FARAZ S. AHMAD, MD, MS
Assistant Professor, Division of Cardiology,
Departments of Medicine (Cardiology) and
Preventive Medicine (Health and Biomedical
Informatics), Center for Health Information
Partnerships, Institute for Public Health and
Medicine, Northwestern University Feinberg
School of Medicine, Chicago, Illinois, USA

LARRY A. ALLEN, MD, MHS
Division of Cardiology, Department of
Medicine, University of Colorado School of
Medicine, Aurora, Colorado, USA

HANNAH ALPHS JACKSON, MD, MHSA
Director, Department of Managed Care,
Northwestern Memorial HealthCare, Assistant
Professor, Department of Surgery, Feinberg
School of Medicine, Northwestern University,
Chicago, Illinois, USA

AAKASH BAVISHI, MD
Fellow, Division of Cardiology, Department
of Medicine, Northwestern University
Feinberg School of Medicine, Chicago, Illinois,
USA

ANKEET S. BHATT, MD, MBA
Division of Cardiovascular Medicine, Brigham
and Women's Hospital, Boston,
Massachusetts, USA

SAUL BLECKER, MD
Assistant Professor, Departments of
Population Health and Medicine, NYU
Grossman School of Medicine, Center for
Healthcare Innovation and Delivery Science,
NYU Langone Health, New York, New York,
USA

THOMAS F. BYRD IV, MD
Instructor, Department of Medicine (Hospital
Medicine), Northwestern University Feinberg
School of Medicine, Chicago, Illinois,
USA

GREGG C. FONAROW, MD
Division of Cardiology, Department of
Medicine, University of California Los Angeles,
Los Angeles, California

ITAI GURVICH, PhD
Professor of Operations Research, Cornell School of Operations Research and Information Engineering, Cornell Tech, New York, New York, USA

BERNARD S. KADOSH, MD
Assistant Professor, Leon H. Charney Division of Cardiology, Department of Medicine, NYU Grossman School of Medicine, New York, New York, USA

STUART D. KATZ, MD
Helen L. and Martin S. Kimmel Professor of Advanced Cardiac Therapeutics, Leon H. Charney Division of Cardiology, Department of Medicine, NYU Grossman School of Medicine, New York, New York, USA

SADIYA S. KHAN, MD, MSc
Assistant Professor, Division of Cardiology, Departments of Medicine and Preventive Medicine, Northwestern University Feinberg School of Medicine, Chicago, Illinois, USA

PRATEETI KHAZANIE, MD, MPH
Division of Cardiology, Department of Medicine, University of Colorado School of Medicine, Aurora, Colorado, USA

ABEL N. KHO, MD
Associate Professor of Medicine, Departments of Medicine (General Internal Medicine and Geriatrics) and Preventive Medicine (Health and Biomedical Informatics), Center for Health Information Partnerships, Institute for Public Health and Medicine, Northwestern University Feinberg School of Medicine, Chicago, Illinois, USA

ORLY LEIVA, MD
Department of Medicine, Brigham and Women's Hospital, Boston, Massachusetts, USA

DAVID M. LIEBOVITZ, MD
Associate Professor of Medicine, Department of Medicine (General Internal Medicine and Geriatrics), Center for Health Information Partnerships, Institute for Public Health and Medicine, Northwestern University Feinberg School of Medicine, Chicago, Illinois, USA

R. KANNAN MUTHARASAN, MD, FACC
Associate Professor of Medicine, Division of Cardiology, Department of Medicine, Northwestern University Feinberg School of Medicine, Chicago, Illinois, USA

IRENE Z. PAN, PharmD
Department of Pharmacy, University of Utah Health, College of Pharmacy, University of Utah, Salt Lake City, Utah, USA

RAVI B. PATEL, MD
Instructor of Medicine, Division of Cardiology, Department of Medicine, Northwestern University Feinberg School of Medicine, Chicago, Illinois, USA

JOHN J. RYAN, MD, MB BCh, BAO
Division of Cardiovascular Medicine, Department of Medicine, University of Utah, Salt Lake City, Utah, USA

SANJIV J. SHAH, MD
Professor of Medicine, Division of Cardiology, Department of Medicine, Northwestern University Feinberg School of Medicine, Chicago, Illinois, USA

JOSEF STEHLIK, MD, MPH
Division of Cardiovascular Medicine, Department of Medicine, University of Utah, Salt Lake City, Utah, USA

MUTHIAH VADUGANATHAN, MD, MPH
Division of Cardiovascular Medicine, Brigham and Women's Hospital, Boston, Massachusetts, USA

JAN ALBERT VAN MIEGHEM, ir, MS, PhD
Harold L. Stuart Professor of Operations Management, Kellogg School of Management at Northwestern University, Evanston, Illinois, USA

JESSICA WALRADT, MS
Manager, Payment Reform, Department of Managed Care, Northwestern Memorial HealthCare, Chicago, Illinois, USA

RAMSEY M. WEHBE, MD
Fellow, Cardiovascular Disease, Division of Cardiology, Department of Medicine, Northwestern University Feinberg School of Medicine, Chicago, Illinois, USA

PETER WOHLFAHRT, MD, PhD
Division of Cardiovascular Medicine, Department of Medicine, University of Utah, Salt Lake City, Utah, USA; Center for Cardiovascular Prevention, Charles University in Prague, First Faculty of Medicine and Thomayer Hospital, Department of Preventive Cardiology, Institute for Clinical and Experimental Medicine, Prague, Czech Republic

Contents

Process improvement begins with the process view: understanding patient care from the patient's point of view. Organizations must also clearly articulate for themselves how they define operational excellence so that the tradeoffs taken in process improvement can be clearly made. Constructing a process map allows application of powerful analytical tools, such as Little's law, which in turn uncovers targets for process improvement from the patient's point of view. Often tradeoffs among process performance metrics, such as quality, cost, time, personalization, and innovation, must be made when deciding upon improvements to be made in certain processes.

Large registries, administrative data, and the electronic health record (EHR) offer opportunities to identify patients with heart failure, which can be used for research purposes, process improvement, and optimal care delivery. Identification of cases is challenging because of the heterogeneous nature of the disease, which encompasses various phenotypes that may respond differently to treatment. The increasing availability of both structured and unstructured data in the EHR has expanded opportunities for cohort construction. This article reviews the current literature on approaches to identification of heart failure, and looks toward the future of machine learning, big data, and phenomapping.

Identifying patients with heart failure at high risk for poor outcomes is important for patient care, resource allocation, and process improvement. Although numerous risk models exist to predict mortality, hospitalization, and patient-reported health status, they are infrequently used for several reasons, including modest performance, lack of evidence to support routine clinical use, and barriers to implementation. Artificial intelligence has the potential to enhance the performance of risk prediction models, but has its own limitations and remains unproved.

Heart failure is a chronic disease with a multitude of different clinical manifestations. Empowering people living with heart failure requires education, support structure, understanding the needs of patients, and reimaging the care delivery systems currently offered to patients. In this article, the authors discuss practical approaches to activate and empower people with heart failure and enable patient-provider dialogue and shared decision making.

The transition from hospitalization to outpatient care is a vulnerable time for patients with heart failure. This requires specific focus on the transitional care period. Here the authors propose a framework to guide process improvement in the transitional care period. The authors extend this framework by (1) examining the role new technology might play in transitional care, and (2) offering practical advice for teams building transitional care programs.

Despite steady progress over the past 3 decades in advancing drug and device therapies to reduce morbidity and mortality in heart failure with reduced ejection fraction, large registries of usual care demonstrate incomplete use of these evidence-based therapies in clinical practice. Potential strategies to improve guideline-directed medical therapy include leveraging non-physician clinicians, solidifying transitions of care, incorporating telehealth solutions, and engaging in comprehensive comorbid disease management via multidisciplinary team structures. These approaches may be particularly relevant in an era of Coronavirus Disease 2019 and associated need for social distancing, further limiting contact with traditional ambulatory clinic settings.

Heart failure (HF) is a growing global epidemic and an increasingly cumbersome burden on health care systems worldwide. As such, optimal management of existing comorbidities in the setting of HF is particularly important to prevent disease progression, reduce HF hospitalizations, and improve quality of life. In this review, the authors address 3 key comorbidities commonly associated with HF: hypertension, atrial fibrillation, and diabetes mellitus. They comprehensively describe the epidemiology, management, and emerging therapies in these 3 disease states as they relate to the overall HF syndrome.

Population health and population health management of patients with heart failure aim to identify all patients with the condition in a population, to characterize and risk stratify subgroups of patients, to improve care delivery by leveraging technology and data so providers can improve care coordination, to engage disease management programs, and to create cost-effective health systems that reduce financial burden on patients and providers. This requires a shift in our treatment paradigm from reactive treatment to proactive primary and secondary prevention. Shifts from fee-for-service to value-based payment models promise to encourage population health.

HEART FAILURE CLINICS

SERIES OF RELATED INTEREST

Cardiology Clinics
http://www.cardiology.theclinics.com/
Cardiac Electrophysiology Clinics
https://www.cardiacep.theclinics.com/
Interventional Cardiology Clinics
https://www.interventional.theclinics.com/

THE CLINICS ARE AVAILABLE ONLINE!
Access your subscription at:
www.theclinics.com

Erratum

An error was made in Volume 16, Issue 3 of *Heart Failure Clinics* on page 349 in "Clinical Application of Stress Echocardiography in Management of Heart Failure" by Kenya Kusunose. **Table 1** should appear as follows.

Table 1
Comparison of advantages and disadvantages between different techniques in stress echocardiography

Methods	Allows for Imaging at Peak Levels	Assessment During Stress	Quantitative Assessment	Ischemic Assessment	Availability	Risk of Complication
Treadmill	No	No	Strong	Strong	Low	Low
Ergometer	Yes	Yes	Strong	Strong	Moderate	Low
6-min walk test	No	No	Weak	Weak	High	Low
Leg-positive pressure	Yes	Yes	Modest	No	Very low	Very low
Leg lifting	Yes	Yes	Weak	No	High	Very low
Hand grip	Yes	Yes	Weak	Weak	Moderate	Very low

Heart Failure Clin 16 (2020) xi
https://doi.org/10.1016/j.hfc.2020.07.001

heartfailure.theclinics.com

Preface

The Critical Need for Process Improvement in Heart Failure

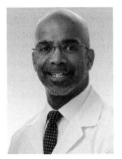

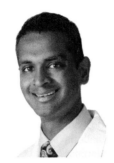

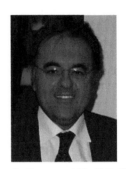

Clyde W. Yancy, MD, MSc, MACC, FAHA, MACP, FHFSA

R. Kannan Mutharasan, MD, FACC

Eduardo Bossone, MD, PhD, FCCP, FESC, FACC

Editors

When we conceived our vision for a contribution to *Heart Failure Clinics* on process improvement in heart failure in mid-2018, we could not have imagined the future we would have to navigate (as of this writing in mid-2020). We have faced 3 major forces that have emphasized that indeed process improvement leading to ideal execution is a much needed skillset if today's challenges are to be overcome and success is to be realized in 2020 and beyond. Those 3 forces have included striking progress in new therapeutics and new approaches in the treatment of heart failure[1]; the glaring exposition of still evident health care disparities brought forward by the pandemic of COVID-19[2,3]; and the heavy weight of racism, including structural racism in medicine,[4] that must now be executed. The triangulation of these compelling forces finds heart failure in the epicenter.

Interposing into this moment an issue on heart failure process improvement may seem at first glance as an imposition, but those of us in the quality improvement space understand that process improvement and the attainment of best quality is race/color/socioeconomic status/sex/gender blind, and with the correct process strategies and performance metrics in place, all persons benefit. This has not however been an easy issue to compose. Our sense of normal has evaporated; we are now in an era where nothing is routine. Even in the absence of a pandemic or in an environment where our awareness of social causes was more quiescent, we would still face an almost unnavigable clinical conundrum—just for heart failure with reduced ejection fraction, there are now 10 approved medical therapeutics, five approved devices, a multitude of accepted care strategies,[5] and an increasingly scrutinized regulatory space still being met with harsh penalties for presumed lapses in care.[6]

We align with those who have remarked that within every crisis lies an opportunity. Thus, we applaud our contributors for seizing this opportunity—even in the midst of this trying moment—and evolving a robust, well-referenced, and deeply grounded approach to process improvement that may restore our current frayed infrastructure and yield a heretofore unimagined victory in the quality of care. We believe the strategies developed in this issue extend far beyond heart failure; we suspect this issue will now serve as a template for other disease entities intent on crafting a path forward.

Our answer to establishing that path forward is simple: process improvement, rooted in pragmatism, is paramount. Our impact on human health is not measured by the elegance of our ideas, but by the fullness of our patients' lives. Can we treat all the right patients at the right time with the correct interventions delivered in the most equitable manner feasible? Process improvement creates the conduit through which the hard-won advances in our laboratories and the successes of our clinical trials flow to people burdened by heart failure. Process improvement creates

Heart Failure Clin 16 (2020) xiii–xv
https://doi.org/10.1016/j.hfc.2020.08.002
1551-7136/20/© 2020 Published by Elsevier Inc.

structure from disorder; emphasizes the patient, regardless of patient characteristics, over the provider; and insists on integration over uncoordinated activity. Building this scaffolding of process improvement helps everyone and especially helps the most vulnerable among us.

In composing this issue, we have invited experts in the field to contribute their latest thinking on diverse topics pertaining to process improvement. You will see from the contents herein that effecting process improvement in modern health care requires a diverse skillset, including understanding operations management principles; harnessing the power of informatics for patient identification, prediction, and records integration; developing a focus on patients and populations while attending to comorbidities; and adapting to new payment models. Not all our contributors are cardiologists; that is for the good. See the economists, data scientists, informatics experts, guideline writing experts, and public policy leaders. This is how we more fully develop the best processes and in turn impact the most patients.

Process improvement work is not easy, and is certainly not glamorous, but it is necessary. We execute the heavy lifting that needs to be done regardless of reward as we understand that good process improvement is the foundational pillar of successful execution. Given the millions of lives and billions of dollars at stake for heart failure alone, we can't miss this opportunity.

We are confident the tools and information in this issue will aid you in your work to improve the care of patients with heart failure. And that through today's multifaceted and challenging lens, this will be the template that will serve as a touchstone for best processes of care in the treatment of heart failure.

Quality of care in heart failure is no longer just about alignment with evidence-based guideline-directed care. In contemporary care we must understand the many dimensions of care and seek every opportunity to optimize outcomes. Process improvement allows us to go well beyond application of guidelines and/or those improvements we can enable with order sets. The incorporation of unique skill sets in informatics, patient-reported outcomes, enabling technologies including electronic health records, and a deeper understanding about population health unlocks significant new potential for process improvement to enhance the life and living experience of those with heart failure. When incorporated with the many iterations of the clinical experience of heart failure including the

surfeit of comorbidities and the ascertainment of risk for poor outcomes, even more opportunities to improve care become evident. Finally, calculating precise value-based assessments and adding best business practices to the model take us well beyond the use of any given indicated medical therapeutic and well into a new era of deep interconnected process improvement. For the challenge that heart failure represents, made so evident during the COVID-19 crisis, these deeper considerations of process improvement are now timely and necessary as we prepare to care for heart failure in the future.

Clyde W. Yancy, MD, MSc, MACC, FAHA, MACP, FHFSA
Division of Cardiology
Northwestern University
Feinberg School of Medicine
676 North Saint Clair Street
Chicago, IL 60611, USA

R. Kannan Mutharasan, MD, FACC
Division of Cardiology
Department of Medicine
Northwestern University
Feinberg School of Medicine
Bluhm Cardiovascular Institute
676 North Saint Clair Street
Chicago, IL 60611, USA

Eduardo Bossone, MD, PhD, FCCP, FESC, FACC
Division of Cardiology
Cardarelli Hospital
Via A. Cardarelli, 9
Naples 80131, Italy

E-mail addresses:
cyancy@nm.org (C.W. Yancy)
kannanm@northwestern.edu (R.K. Mutharasan)
ebossone@hotmail.com (E. Bossone)

REFERENCES

1. Vaduganathan M, Claggett BL, Jhund PS, et al. Estimating lifetime benefits of comprehensive disease-modifying pharmacological therapies in patients with heart failure with reduced ejection fraction: a comparative analysis of three randomised controlled trials. Lancet 2020;396(10244):121–8. https://doi.org/10.1016/S0140-6736(20)30748-0.
2. Yancy CW. COVID-19 and African Americans. JAMA 2020. https://doi.org/10.1001/jama.2020.6548.
3. Bhala N, Curry G, Martineau AR, et al. Sharpening the global focus on ethnicity and race in the time of COVID-19. Lancet 2020;395(10238):1673–6. https://doi.org/10.1016/S0140-6736(20)31102-8.

4. Yancy CW. Academic medicine and black lives matter: time for deep listening. JAMA 2020. https://doi.org/10.1001/jama.2020.12532.

5. Takeda A, Martin N, Taylor RS, et al. Disease management interventions for heart failure. Cochrane Database Syst Rev 2019;(1):CD002752. https://doi.org/10.1002/14651858.CD002752.pub4.

6. Wadhera RK, Vaduganathan M, Jiang GY, et al. Performance in federal value-based programs of hospitals recognized by the American Heart Association and American College of Cardiology for high-quality heart failure and acute myocardial infarction care. JAMA Cardiol 2020. https://doi.org/10.1001/jamacardio.2020.0001.

Introduction

Process Improvement in Heart Failure

If you can't describe what you are doing as a process, you don't know what you're doing.
—W. Edwards Deming

We are delighted to see this much-needed series on "Process Improvement in Heart Failure." The goal of health care is to help people live longer and better lives. The extent to which health care delivery accomplishes this overall goal represents the quality of that care. Unfortunately, the quality of care delivery in the United States, particularly for chronic conditions like heart failure (HF), lags behind many other countries and has marked gaps, variations, and disparities.[1] Two decades ago, 2 landmark works from Institute of Medicine brought attention to the need for process improvement: *To Err Is Human: Building a Safer Health System* (1999)[2] and *Crossing the Quality Chasm: A New Health System for the 21st Century* (2001).[3] The latter called for a fundamental change in the health care delivery system through a complete redesign of patient-provider relationships and revised patient care processes, leading to improved health care outcomes. It fundamentally recognized that quality improvement cannot solely rely upon demanding that individual clinicians "do better"—quality problems are systems problems that require systems solutions.

This call to action for "Process Improvement in HF" is as timely as ever, as the care of patients with HF is, in many ways, at an inflection point. Diagnostic biomarkers, imaging, and genetics help us identify HF better than ever. In HF with reduced ejection fraction there are now a plethora of medicines and pacing devices that work additively to improve cardiac structure and performance. For the first time we are seeing therapies that may help HF patients with relatively preserved left ventricular ejection fraction. Our ability to monitor patients' hemodynamics, activity, and adherence has increased exponentially, and in ways that may translate to meaningful actions. And, our ability to coordinate all this care through information technology is finally achieving meaningful use. Quite simply, we can do more than ever to help improve care and clinical outcomes patients with HF. Yet, despite all of that, the epidemic of HF is as challenging as ever. Once disease is present, most patients are managed rather than cured. Polypharmacy, multimorbidity, frailty, and health illiteracy all complicate treatment. Gaps in prescribing, dose intensification, and adherence leave the vast majority of patients on suboptimal treatment regimens. And, siloed care delivery, electronic health records designed around billing, and opaque payment models all act to depersonalize patients while burning out clinicians. Without a serious commitment to improving processes of care, many of the scientific advances now available to patients with HF will be lost.[4] It is time to double down on process improvement.

Much has been written about process, primarily from the business disciplines. Within health care, process improvement is the framework for how to systematically improve the ways care is delivered to patients.[5] The Donabedian model of quality is a helpful construct for approaching quality improvement. It describes 3 main domains of quality: structure, process, and outcomes.[6] Health systems provide infrastructure. Patients care about their outcomes. And clinicians and other health care providers mostly have control over process (ie, what we do). Thus, a detailed look at process improvement in HF is highly relevant to anyone actively delivering care to people with HF.

In the longitudinal care of patients with HF, innumerable processes are required in the delivery of care. Prevention, screening, determining cause, initiation and intensification of guideline-directed medical therapies, efficient monitoring and imaging, appropriate use of devices, and timely transition to end-of-life care are all complex care processes that span time, locations, and providers. These processes have characteristics that can be measured, analyzed, improved, and controlled. In parallel, an exponentially growing body of medical research and clinical evidence continues to refine best practices. The tools of process improvement bring operational processes and medical evidence together through guidelines, data standards, quality metrics and performance measures, national registries and benchmarking, policy, and payment. These are all highly relevant to the care of patients with HF and fit into a comprehensive cycle of activities that work to define, measure, and ultimately promote quality HF care.[7]

Heart Failure Clin 16 (2020) xvii–xix
https://doi.org/10.1016/j.hfc.2020.08.003
1551-7136/20/© 2020 Published by Elsevier Inc.

The foundation of any quality improvement effort is measurement. Peter Drucker famously said, "If you can't measure it, you can't improve it." Without systematic assessment and evaluation, the quality of care is difficult to know, and the targets for intervention are unclear. Participation in national clinical registries/quality improvement programs offers a method for accurately assessing processes and outcomes and offers feedback on how individual hospital and clinician practices compare with their peers through benchmarking performance against aggregate national or similar hospital outcomes following adjustment for case mix. These quality improvement programs also help share and disseminate best practices and process improvement techniques that can be tailored and implemented locally.

Process improvement can work. Perhaps the most notable example of a national clinical registries/quality improvement program in HF is the American Heart Association's Get With The Guidelines (GWTG).[8] GWTG-HF is an in-hospital program for improving care by promoting consistent adherence to the latest scientific treatment guidelines. Hospitals participating in GWTG-HF have been able to achieve and sustain high rates of use of the full set of guideline-directed medical therapies, a high level of conformity with device therapy, along with provision of HF patient education.[9] With GWTG-HF, improvements in care quality have been attained in hospitals teaching and nonteaching, large and small, rural and urban, from all regions in the United States. Variations in care between hospitals have been reduced over time, and age, sex, race-ethnicity disparities in HF care quality have been reduced or entirely eliminated with GWTG-HF participation. Quality of care and clinical outcomes for participating hospitals have been shown to be superior to that of comparable hospitals not participating. Numerous published studies demonstrate the program's success in achieving significant patient outcome improvements. On the ambulatory side, historically the Registry to Improve the Use of Evidence-Based Heart Failure Therapies in the Outpatient Setting (IMPROVE HF) prospectively tested a multidimensional practice-specific performance improvement intervention on the use of guideline-recommended therapies for HF in outpatient cardiology and multispecialty practices.[10] There were substantial improvements in guideline-directed medical and device therapy in eligible HF patients without contraindications, reduced practice-based variation in care, and equitable improvement in care quality by sex/race-ethnicity. The resulting greater conformity

with guideline-directed care was associated with lower risk of 24-month all-cause mortality. Currently, the American College of Cardiology's PINNACLE Registry is cardiology's largest outpatient registry, capturing data on hypertension, coronary artery disease, atrial fibrillation, and HF.[11]

But models like GWTG-HF, IMPROVE-HF, and PINNACLE are rare and have not been promulgated well. Only a quarter of US hospitals participate in GWTG-HF, and only 700 or so cardiology practices submit data to PINNACLE. There are numerous examples of single-center process improvement initiatives, but overwhelmingly they have been not been sustainable or scalable. Internationally, quality improvement efforts in HF have been infrequent to date, and most efforts have reported no to limited success in improving care quality. As present, the majority of HF patients in the United States and globally are still cared for in settings without the benefit of robust quality improvement systems being deployed.

The way forward is taking shape. The burden of high-cost, low-quality care combined with a growing population with chronic comorbid conditions like HF is forcing greater attention on shifting from volume-based to value-based payment.[12] The Affordable Care Act and other major health care legislative acts have had an important impact on the care of HF patients through the regulation of the health insurance industry, expansion of access to health care, and the creation of several alternative payment models. However, the benefits of value-based and alternative payment models such as the Hospital Readmissions Reduction Program and bundled payment programs for HF outcomes are less clear, and controversy exists regarding whether some of these programs may even worsen outcomes while they cut costs.[13] Value is quality over cost. In the HF space, it is hoped, we will see the bulk of health reform efforts focus on improving quality rather than merely reducing cost.

Furthermore, one of the most effective ways to "treat" HF is to prevent it. There are effective therapies and strategies that can markedly lower the risk of incident HF, such as treatment of high blood pressure to optimal levels, use of sodium glucose cotransporter 2 inhibitors in patients with type 2 diabetes mellitus, and prevention of myocardial infarction. Process improvement systems need to be broadly implemented with the goal of preventing HF.

It is estimated that if process improvement for HF treatment were implemented, optimally more than 100,000 lives a year of HF patients in United States could be saved.[14] We consider that worth the effort. Therefore, we believe that this *Heart Failure Clinics* issue is an important call to action for process improvement in HF care delivery. The following series of articles not only focuses attention on how to use new therapies but also optimizes best use of medical therapies, devices, disease management, and shared decision making. Let's get to work implementing process improvement!

Larry A. Allen, MD, MHS
Division of Cardiology
Department of Medicine
University of Colorado School of Medicine
Asnchutz Medical Campus
12631 East 17th Avenue
Academic Office One, #7019, Mailstop B130
Aurora, CO 80045, USA

Gregg C. Fonarow, MD
Division of Cardiology
Department of Medicine
University of California Los Angeles
100 Medical Plaza Driveway, Suite 630
Los Angeles, CA 90095, USA

E-mail addresses:
larry.allen@cuanschutz.edu (L.A. Allen)
GFonarow@mednet.ucla.edu (G.C. Fonarow)

REFERENCES

1. Dartmouth Atlas Project. Available at: http://www.dartmouthatlas.org/. Accessed January 10, 2020.
2. Institute of Medicine. To err is human: building a safer health system. 1999. Available at: http://www.nationalacademies.org/hmd/~/media/Files/Report%20Files/1999/To-Err-is-Human/To%20Err%20is%20Human%201999%20%20report%20brief.pdf. Accessed January 10, 2020.
3. Crossing the quality chasm: a new health system for the 21st century. 2001. Available at: http://www.nationalacademies.org/hmd/~/media/Files/Report%20Files/2001/Crossing-the-Quality-Chasm/Quality%20Chasm%202001%20%20report%20brief.pdf. Accessed January 10, 2020.
4. Green SJ, Butler J, Albert NM, et al. Medical therapy for heart failure with reduced ejection fraction: the CHAMP-HF registry. J Am Coll Cardiol 2018;72(4):351–66.
5. Agency for Healthcare Research and Quality, Practice Facilitation Handbook. Available at: https://www.ahrq.gov/ncepcr/tools/pf-handbook/mod4.html. Accessed January 10, 2020.
6. Ayanian JZ, Markel H. Donabedian's lasting framework for health care quality. N Engl J Med 2016;375:205–7.
7. Califf RM, Harrington RA, Madre LK, et al. Curbing the cardiovascular disease epidemic: aligning industry, government, payers, and academics. Health Aff (Millwood) 2007;26:62–74.
8. Get With the Guidelines. Available at: https://www.heart.org/en/professional/quality-improvement/get-with-the-guidelines/get-with-the-guidelines-heart-failure. Accessed January 10, 2020.
9. Ellrodt AG, Fonarow GC, Schwamm LH, et al. Synthesizing lessons learned from Get With The Guidelines: the value of disease-based registries in improving quality and outcomes. Circulation 2013;128(22):2447–60.
10. Fonarow GC, Albert NM, Curtis AB, et al. Improving evidence-based care for heart failure in outpatient cardiology practices: primary results of the Registry to Improve the Use of Evidence-Based Heart Failure Therapies in the Outpatient Setting (IMPROVE HF). Circulation 2010;122(6):585–96.
11. PINNACLE. Available at: https://cvquality.acc.org/NCDR-Home/registries/outpatient-registries/pinnacle-registry. Accessed January 10, 2020.
12. Wolfe JD, Joynt Maddox KE. Heart failure and the affordable care act: past, present, and future. JACC Heart Fail 2019;7(9):737–45.
13. Psotka MA, Fonarow GC, Allen LA, et al. The hospital readmissions reduction program: nationwide perspectives and recommendations. JACC Heart Fail 2020;8(1):1–11.
14. Fonarow GC, Hernandez AF, Solomon SD, et al. Potential mortality reduction with optimal implementation of angiotensin receptor neprilysin inhibitor therapy in heart failure. JAMA Cardiol 2016;1(6):714–7.

Approaching Process Improvement

Itai Gurvich, PhD[a], R. Kannan Mutharasan, MD, FACC[b],
Jan Albert Van Mieghem, ir, MS, PhD[c],*

KEYWORDS

- Process improvement • Heart failure • Health care operations

KEY POINTS

- A process view of patient care, focusing attention on the patient rather than on the system or the strategy, is an important tool for approaching process improvement, particularly for complex conditions like heart failure.
- Process improvement drives operational excellence. In the health care context, this may be defined as the ability to deliver value to patients efficiently.
- Process mapping and flow time analysis are quantitative approaches to identifying process waste and focusing process improvement efforts.
- Process improvement requires considering personalization and standardization. Personalized care can be delivered in a standardized way. Although personalization increases complexity, standardizing the workflow controls cost and quality.
- Starting and sustaining process improvement requires communicating objectives, engaging stakeholders, tracking metrics, and embracing the continuous nature of the process of process improvement itself.

Before we discuss how to start and manage process improvement, let us review what a process is and introduce 3 perspectives to describe processes.

WHAT IS A PROCESS AND A PROCESS VIEW?

Think about the last time you went as a patient to a hospital or as a customer to a coffee shop to order and enjoy a drink or a snack. How would you describe your interaction with the various caregivers or employees? What did these caregivers do, and how did they perform the work?

A good way to describe this is by thinking about how you, as a patient or customer, flow through the various steps of the process. When you view an organization through this lens, we say that we adopt a process view. If you think about the coffee shop, you might say that you are adopting a process view of the coffee shop. This process view is the start of understanding, analyzing, and improving any operation.

A process is a transformation of inputs into outputs. At the highest system level, the transformation could be a black box. However, in order to analyze and improve a process, you need to "open up" the black box and describe the different steps inside the process. These steps are activities and buffers. Activities are the steps whereby work gets done, whereas buffers are instances whereby flow units are waiting. Buffers often also are handoffs between 2 different activities whereby collaboration is important.

Funding: The authors received no funding.
[a] Cornell School of Operations Research and Information Engineering, Cornell Tech, 2 West Loop Road, New York, NY 10044, USA; [b] Northwestern University Feinberg School of Medicine, 676 North Saint Clair Street, Arkes Pavilion, Suite 6-071, Chicago, IL 60611, USA; [c] Kellogg School of Management at Northwestern University, GLOBAL HUB 2211 Campus Dr, Evanston, IL 60201, USA
* Corresponding author.
E-mail address: VanMieghem@northwestern.edu

Heart Failure Clin 16 (2020) 369–377
https://doi.org/10.1016/j.hfc.2020.06.001

You should ask 4 key questions when adopting a process view of an organization. Let us look at these questions in the context of the discharge process for a patient who is hospitalized for heart failure (**Fig. 1**).

First, you need to ask *what the process boundaries are*. In other words, what are the inputs and outputs? For the discharge process, the inputs include the patient, laboratory results, and any other entities needed to complete discharge. The outputs are a treated patient with a disposition plan together with perhaps a letter to the primary care physician and any medications.[1,2] Inputs and outputs thus are typically multidimensional.

Second, *ask what is the flow unit* or the unit of analysis that you want to focus on is. Then, attach yourself to the flow unit and record all the process steps that touch the flow unit. In the discharge process, the workflow would be the various medical workup and treatment steps through which a patient and laboratory results flow. In parallel to the discharge process runs the disposition process. Several interactions among the various activities give rise to a network, which captures the primary workflow depicted using a typical process flow diagram. Activities are represented by rectangles, and buffers are represented by triangles. Any lack of synchronization among activities, such as medical treatment and disposition, may lead to waiting in buffers.

The third question to ask is *who does the work*. In other words, what are the human and capital resources needed to execute each activity? Processing resources fall into 2 categories: human resources (various types of caregivers, administrators, technicians, and so forth) and capital assets (beds, patient rooms, operating rooms, waiting rooms, imaging equipment, and so forth).

Last, ask yourself *what information is required* to perform each activity. Where does this information come from? This information can come from communication among resources and patients, as well as from electronic health records and other planning or execution software.

In summary, a process is a transformation of inputs into outputs using a well-structured sequence of activities and buffers. This process view (as depicted by a process flow chart) shows how work is done in an organization. This process view is customer-centric and highlights the purpose of the organization: how is value created for its customers.

Adopting this process view (and a process flow chart depicting the sequence of activities) is the start of understanding, analyzing, and improving how value is delivered to the process customer (the patient). However, in the authors' experience, many organizations tend to adopt a resource view and focus on who performs the work: this would result in a flow chart depicting the various types of human and capital resources (and a jumbled flow of how patients go from 1 resource to the next, often using the physical layout of rooms and facilities). Theoretically, the resource view is the "dual" representation of the process view (boxes represent a resource vs boxes represent an activity). However, it is internally focused and highlights the resources needed for the value creation, rather than focus on the patient flow.

In addition to the process and resource views, it is strategically important to consider a "competency view," which describes what kind of work

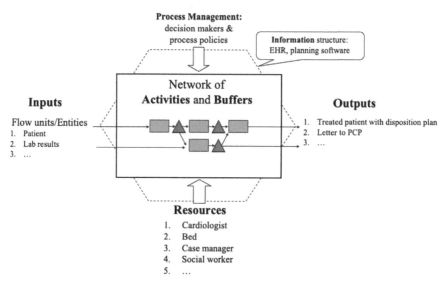

Fig. 1. A process view of discharge. EHR, electronic health record; PCP, primary care physician.

the organization excels at. Although often difficult, one must rank the importance, and the organization's capability, of delivering (i) quality of outcomes, (ii) quality of experience (for the patient or the employees), (iii) timeliness, (iv) cost, and (v) variety of services offered and their personalization. For example, the key competency for an emergency department is the ability to handle any patient type in a timely manner. Of course, cost and quality matter too, but it is unrealistic to expect the same quality from a specialist handling a very narrow set of issues as one would expect from a generalist. Strategic thinking means clearly acknowledging tradeoffs, even if this is uncomfortable or difficult. Therefore, a competency view is strategically important because it sets the priorities to be considered when tradeoffs must be made and how performance should be measured.

WHAT IS PROCESS IMPROVEMENT AND OPERATIONAL EXCELLENCE?

Think about the strategic goals of your organization: how do you prioritize the importance of *quality, price, time, variety and personalization, innovation* in the patient value proposition? How does this relate to process improvement and the often-stated aspiration of operational excellence? What does it even mean to become operationally excellent? Even though there is no simple answer to that question, we propose 3 perspectives of operational excellence.

The first is a strategic perspective of operational excellence. You need to structure your operating system so that your operational competencies are aligned with your value proposition. Your operating system is the processes and resources that you use to create a product or deliver a service. For example, the FedEx operating system is structured to deliver an overnight service, whereas the US Postal Service is structured to provide a slower but more affordable service. Their operating systems are structured differently because each promises something different to their customers. Similarly, an emergency department (whose strategic priorities are timeliness and variety) must be structured differently than a dialysis department (given that most of its services are homogeneous and predictable, its strategic priorities are cost and quality).

The hallmark of good strategy is the alignment of the means with the goals. In the case of operations, the means is the operating system and the goal is how you create value for your customers. FedEx promises fast, reliable delivery and is structured to have an overnight service. Strategic alignment is a requirement for operational excellence

but not a sufficient condition by itself to ensure it. You may have the right process steps and resources, but you may still have waste in your execution.

Next is the financial perspective of operational excellence. You are operationally excellent if you maximize the net present value of your operation. This means that you have optimized the value your operation creates. You can calculate this by subtracting the cost of your operation from the benefit to your customers. This quantitative perspective allows you to come up with prescriptions: for example, what are your optimal capacity and your optimal inventory to maximize the value of your organization?

However, we often operate in competitive markets, and so we must also consider our competition. This brings us to the competitive perspective of operational excellence. You are operationally excellent if no rival can provide the same value proposition at a lower cost, or, equivalently, more value at the same cost. For example, your company needs to provide more flexibility and faster service to your customers at the same cost as your rival or provide the same level of service and flexibility at a lower cost.

If you can achieve this, you are on the *efficient frontier* and no other rival surpasses you. The *efficient frontier* is defined by all the organizations that are not being outcompeted by a rival.

Bringing all 3 perspectives of operational excellence together impacts the entire organization. It requires alignment of the operating system with the management infrastructure as well as the mindset and behavior of all the employees of the organization. Overall, operational excellence requires strategic alignment as well as maximizing your value so that you are on the efficient frontier.

Given this insight into what it *actually* means to be operationally excellent, we next proceed with answering 2 questions:

1. How close is your organization to achieving operational excellence? (Assessment, evaluation)
2. How and where can we improve our process? (Improvement, optimization)

PROCESS METRICS: EVALUATION AND IMPROVEMENT

Having mapped your process, by following the flow unit and recording the steps and the resources performing, you can turn to a structured evaluation and improvement of your process. Improvement depends on how you have defined operational excellence for your process.

We must start with 3 key process metrics: flow time (how much time does it take, on average, to process a patient from beginning to end of this process), throughput (the average flow rate = the average number of patients served per hour), and the census of patients (or the "inventory" of patients = the average number of patients in the system). Their structured definition will reveal avenues to improve upon them. We will also introduce Little's law: a powerful rule that governs the relationship between these 3 metrics.

A toy example will be useful for illustration. For a deeper treatment, we refer to Anupindi and colleagues.[3] We use cardiology-relevant terms to make the example easier to place in context. Take a process with 5 numbered activities. Activity A can be thought of representing the first step of diagnosis and treatment. Activities B and C represent the treatment, while activities D and E represent the disposition planning process. Activity F represents the discharge task. The example is as follows.

Flow time refers to the average time it takes a unit to flow through the process from entry to exit: time spent in activities + time spent in buffer = processing (or activity) time + waiting time. Flow time metrics are common in health care: time until appointment for outpatient settings, and door-to-doctor in the emergency room (ER) are only 2 examples. Not all of the flow time is value added. Some of the flow time is spent on value-adding activities (an examination, an MRI) but some, often nonnegligible, is spent on waiting for resources to become available to serve the unit of flow. We separate flow time into value-added time and delays. Let us pretend at first that we have infinite resources. In that case, the time that a flow unit, a patient, spends in the process depicted in **Fig. 2** is composed of the sum of processing times in the various steps/activities the unit has to undergo. This is in this case 6 hours (summing up the six 1-hour activities). Then, the patient's *theoretic flow time* is 6 hours.

This flow time can be improved if some activities are performed in parallel. Medical treatment and disposition for a heart failure patient are generally separate activities (**Fig. 3**). Performing these activities in parallel will improve the flow time. In this redesigned process, a patient is discharged when both treatment and disposition are completed. Thus, in general, the theoretic flow time is determined by the so-called critical path. This is the longest path in the network of activities from entry to exit. In this case, the longer path is the treatment path, which takes $A + B + C + F = 4$ hours > 3.5 hours $= A + D + E + F$. Because of variability in processing times, the actual flow times (in the absence of delays) will be typically longer than the maximum of the 2 paths averages. Nevertheless, this simple calculation provides a lower bound.

This definition of theoretic flow time also uncovers ways to *improve* it. It helps identifying focal points for effort. The most valuable improvements are those that shorten the critical path. In moving the disposition activities D and E off the critical path and paralleling them with treatment, we have shortened the critical path that now has only activities A, B, C, and F. If precedence requirements prevent such parallelization, then it is useful to focus on shortening activities on the critical path itself.

The second component of flow time is the delay accrued waiting for resources to become available. It is important to distinguish between waiting that adds value (waiting for the effect of a medication; we would think of this as an activity whereby the resource is only the bed), and waiting that does not add value (when all results are ready and the physician is still busy with another patient).

Delays are a product of the interaction of load (the average utilization of the resource = the fraction of time the resource has to work to process all arriving inputs) and the variability of the inputs (of the arrival process itself and of the input processing times). If, on average, 2 patients per hour require the attention of the cardiologist, who has to spend 25 minutes with each, then the cardiologist's load/utilization is 50 minutes/60 minutes of availability per hour = $\frac{5}{6}$. It seems intuitive that the greater the load, the more patients will have to wait. Indeed, it is obvious and true that if the load exceeds 100%, delays are unavoidable. Aligning capacity with average demand is the key step to avoid this; see discussion of capacity later.

Unavoidable delays can occur even at loads less than 100%. This is because of variability. In

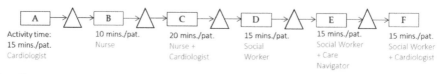

Fig. 2. A baseline process.

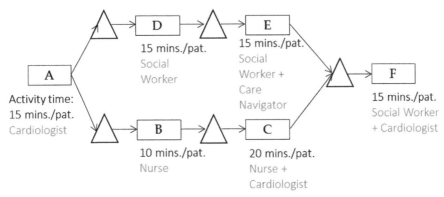

Fig. 3. A redesigned process with parallel processing.

our example, the load is $\frac{5}{6}$ and hence less than 100%. If a patient arrives exactly every 30 minutes, requiring exactly 25 minutes of care, no patient would have to wait. However, if the processing time is sometimes 40 minutes and sometimes 10 minutes (still 25 minutes on average), some patients will have to wait. **Fig. 4** captures the way that load/utilization and variability interact. For a given utilization, the average delay increases with variability. For a given variability level, the delay increases in an exponential fashion with utilization: as utilization approaches 100%, the delay increases substantially. In the presence of *any* variability, it is crucial to have a significant capacity buffer if one were to have short delays. High utilization has an unavoidable effect on delays.

The graph reveals the levers for delay improvement. One can decrease utilization: reducing patient processing time from 25 to 20 minutes would reduce utilization from $\frac{5}{6}$ to $\frac{2}{3}$. Adding a cardiologist would reduce the load because the input of 2 patients per hour is now split between the 2 so that the utilization of each is $(\frac{5}{6})/2 = 5/12$. The other lever is reducing variability in processing time. Clinical pathways, for example, are a mechanism through which variability is reduced.

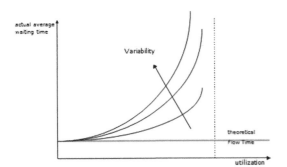

Fig. 4. The fundamental relationship between delay, resource utilization, and variability in throughput and activity times.

Throughput and Capacity

The throughput is the average number of patients that our cardiology process handles per unit of time. In general process terms, it is the number of flow units that enter the process per unit of time. Assuming that the units do not accumulate indefinitely or disappear inside the process, in the long run, the number of units that enter should be the same as those that exit. Throughput is the minimum of the input/demand (we will not process more patients than those that arrive) and the capacity of the process (the maximal number of patients the process *can* handle per unit of time).

It turns out that if we know the throughput and the flow time, we actually also know the census.

Census and Inventory

Although the word inventory is typically associated with items rather than humans, in the context of process analysis, it refers to any flow units that are in the process. In health care, if our flow unit is a patient, then inventory refers to the patients within the process boundaries. It thus can measure the patient census in the ER or in the cardiology ward. If our flow unit is an image, the inventory may also refer to the queue of images waiting for a review by a radiologist.

The fundamental Little's law (named after John D.C. Little, who set it on mathematical footing[4]) states that inventory, flow time, and throughput are related:

Average inventory = throughput * average flow time

For example, if the average arrival of patient to the ER (throughput) is 240 per day, and patients spend on average 3 hours = 1/8 days in the ER, then the number of patients in the ER is 240*1/8 = 30 on average. Although this relationship holds mathematically in the long run (as an average over many days), it empirically also holds remarkably well over shorter horizons.

The importance of this law is that it reveals that (i) we can predict delays from looking at historical census and throughput data. Alternatively, we can predict census from flow time and throughput data; and (ii) that, to improve census, one must either reduce throughput or flow time (so that their product decreases). *In short, there are only 2 degrees of freedom among the 3 fundamental process metrics:* throughput, flow time, and inventory (census)*: once 2 are known, then so is the third.*

Recall that throughput is the minimum of demand and process capacity. The latter is now considered.

Capacity is the maximal sustainable number of patients the process can serve. It is expressed as a rate: patients per hour, patients per shift, and so forth. Capacity is the upper bound on throughput. If demand exceeds this number, some patients must be rejected. Ultimately, limitations on throughput (ie, process capacity) result from limitations on the resources that perform the activities. Therefore, to determine and improve capacity, we must adopt a resource view, and we summarize our calculations in **Table 1**.

Let us first consider the capacity of each resource in isolation, ignoring the coordination between resources. Take, for example, the cardiologist in our basic example. How many patients could the cardiologist process (assuming this is the only activity the cardiologist performs)? Let us assume that the cardiologist spends 50 minutes per patient (15 minutes in each of activities A and F and 20 minutes in activity C). To further simplify the example, let us assume that all of this work is done on 1 day, the arithmetic still holds if the work is broken up. Because the cardiologist has 60 minutes in an hour, the cardiologist can see at most $60/50 = 1.2$ patients on an average hour, or 6 patients every 5 hours. This is the cardiologist's capacity. We can repeat

this for each of the resources in the network, leading to a table such as **Table 1**. The resource with the lowest resource capacity is the slowest resource, also called the *bottleneck resource.* The bottleneck resource is the constraint on the process throughput: even if other resources improve their capacity (eg, even if the nurse doubles the speed), the bottleneck resource (eg, the cardiologist) is still going to be the slowest and constrain the number of patients that this process can handle. It should be clear that regardless of how well we coordinate work, because every patient has to see the cardiologist, we cannot see more than 1.2 patients per hour. This calculation gives the upper bound.

Evaluating process capacity by identifying the bottleneck resources presents us with levers on how to improve process capacity. Just as the critical path is the focus of attention to improve theoretic flow time, so is the bottleneck the focus of attention for improvement of capacity. We can obviously do this by reducing activity times (from 15 minutes for final discharge to say 10 minutes = this would equate the load of the cardiologist with that of social worker, increasing the process capacity to 1.33 patients per hour). We can also consider adding a resource. Adding a cardiologist would translate into the cardiologists' capacity (as a group) of 2.4 patients per hour. However, after any process change, one must reidentify the bottleneck because the bottleneck can shift. If we add a cardiologist in our example, the process capacity will not double because the bottleneck then shifts to the social worker, which will constrain the capacity to 1.33 patients per hour. Thus, when the performance of a bottleneck is improved, another resource might become a bottleneck. These improvements thus must be made incrementally, observing when the bottleneck shifts.

We can also consider redesigning the process activities. For example, if we can split the

Table 1
Theoretic capacity calculations

Resource	Unit Load (Time/Job), min/Patient	Resource Capacity			Process Capacity, Patient/h	Resource Utilization at Capacity
		Unit Capacity, Patient/h	No. of Units	Total, Patient/h		
Cardiologist	50	1.2	1	1.2	1.2	$(1.2) \div (1.2) = 100\%$
Nurse	30	2	1	2	1.2	$(1.2) \div (2) = 60\%$
Social worker	45	1.33	1	1.33	1.2	$(1.2) \div (1.33) = 90\%$
Care navigator	15	4	1	4	1.2	$(1.2) \div (4) = 30\%$

discharge activity F into 2 subactivities F1 and F2, taking 5 and 10 minutes, respectively, and assign F1 to the nurse and social worker (while F2 still requires the cardiologist and social workers), we would be removing 5 minutes of the cardiologist's load. The cardiologist and social worker would now be both bottlenecks each having a load of 45 minutes per patient, increasing the process capacity to 1.33 patients per hour.

Taking a Step Back

Recall the question that opens this article, "How do you prioritize the importance of *quality, cost, time, variety and personalization, innovation* in the patient value proposition?" The cost per patient can include the variable cost of processing an activity (eg, the cost of blood draw for 1 patient) and fixed process costs that can be independent of the activity levels or throughput (eg, beds and rooms have a fixed cost component that is independent of their utilization or the number of patients served). Process capacity depends on assigned resources and thus often has a fixed cost component: if one can increase the process capacity while keeping the assigned resources unchanged, then the cost per patient served is reduced. Time, as a competitive dimension, is formalized in our process via the flow time, which includes value-adding activities and waiting time.

Quality

Quality of care is a broad and loaded term. To operationalize it, we must be specific and precise. When evaluating the quality of a process, we should ask how well it performs relative to *what it is designed to deliver*. Some processes have unavoidable variable outputs. A coin is "designed" to fall on Head half of the time and on Tail the other half. For example, suppose we design a follow-up cardiology clinic so that 80% of discharged patients can be seen within 7 days of discharge.[5] On some weeks, we will achieve the target and, because of variability, it is unavoidable that we will occasionally miss this target. The question is how frequently this will happen. The less variable the process, the less frequent these events and, we will say, the more *capable* the process. This process would be a 6-sigma process if the event of missing the target is as unlikely as an outcome that is 6 standard deviations away from the mean. Improvement, within this view, is about either moving the mean (doing better on average than 80%) or reducing the variability so that we meet the target more often.

Given the designed capability of the process, we must monitor the process to ensure that it continues to perform as planned. In the simple coin example, we would maintain that the coin is unbiased as long as, informally speaking, the Heads and Tails appear in equal proportions. However, if we have a long sequence of tosses over which this balance is broken, we might suspect that something happened to the coin. Statistical process control is the set of tools to monitor processes and trigger alarms when the observed variability exceeds the expected variability of the process. If such an alarm sounds, one should investigate whether the process has deviated from its design.

Statistical process control is also useful in the context of process improvement and redesign. Consider, for example, **Fig. 5**, taken from a case study of an intervention aimed to reduce door-to-doctor time in an emergency department.[6] Because there is variability in the door-to-door time (also postintervention), statistical process control is used to verify that the performance observed shortly after the intervention represents a real change to the process rather than random outcomes. In this way, statistical process control is also used to verify that process changes had the intended effects.[4]

Personalization Versus Standardization

Personalized care is important to the patient, whereas standardized work is important for ensuring quality and improvement. To understand the connection and the difference between personalization and standardization, let us first clarify and define both concepts. Personalization means that the product or the service (ie, the process) is tailored to the person (patient). Standardized work means that each activity has a clearly documented set of instructions that is followed by each resource that executes that activity. The obvious need for standardized work is to "bring the process in control" (ie, reduce and maintain variability) and to set a benchmark against which process improvements can be validated (similar to a random control trial: the standardized work is the control, the improvement is the trial or experiment).

Although personalization adds challenges and complexity, the key insight is that operational excellence can provide personalized service with standardized work. This is similar to how some automobile manufacturers can provide vehicles with bespoke features on the same assembly line.

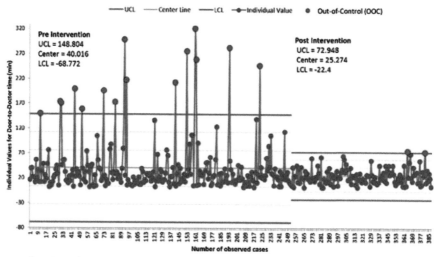

Fig. 5. The use of statistical process control to verify the effects of process redesign. LCL, lower control limit; UCL, upper control limit.

Similarly, although patients often require different care, health care processes and/or subprocesses are often standardized. Whereas what happens *in* a consult with a cardiologist may be specific to the patient, the path leading *to* this consult (appointment scheduling, check-in, vitals) and after this consult may be common to most patients. Of course, there are limits to the personalization that can be provided with a largely common process flow. For example, the input (patients) to an ER is so variable and unpredictable that care is not (indeed cannot be) fully standardized across patients. It is inefficient in the context of emergency care to have different ERs for different disease groups. In contrast, several cancer clinics have separated their ambulatory chemotherapy from other cancer treatment processes. Assigning different segments of patients to separate processes allows for greater standardization, greater focus with less complexity, and possibly increased efficiency.

The operational and financial challenge with providing different processes is clear if we put them in the context of the operational metrics we discuss later. We have seen how variability of inputs and processing times affects delays. Standardizing care often will mean reducing this variability, a result also of the reduction of coordination and resource-movement delays, and hence reducing delays. However, providing various services by 1 shared set of resources can also decrease capacity because equipment (and personnel) will incur setup and changeover times (either mental or physical, as in the setting up of an operating room between 2 different types of surgeries). In other words, personalization introduces operational tradeoffs. Lean operations, which we connect to next, are about consistently trying to reduce these tradeoffs.

HOW TO GET STARTED WITH PROCESS IMPROVEMENT AND HOW TO SUSTAIN IT?

Having discussed how to adopt a process view of your organizational unit and to analyze it, we conclude with 4 guidelines to start process improvement and, perhaps more importantly, sustain it:

1. Communicate your objectives clearly and often. What exactly are you aspiring to improve: quality (at a certain activity, of outcomes, of experience?), responsiveness (patient access, patient flow time?), throughput, cost? These improvement priorities should be aligned with the strategic priorities of the entire organization. This implies that executive support, if not leadership, is essential for the improvement process to be effective, to be implemented, and to last.
2. Engage and empower all stakeholders in the process. Holding daily huddles at the start of a shift can be very effective, especially when coupled with the next guideline.
3. Track metrics and visualize them. Having decided on the strategic improvement objectives, track the associated key performance metrics and prioritize them accordingly. Huddles around a board of the key performance indicators, including new action items, ideas, or people to be recognized, as well as projected savings is a powerful tool for process improvement.

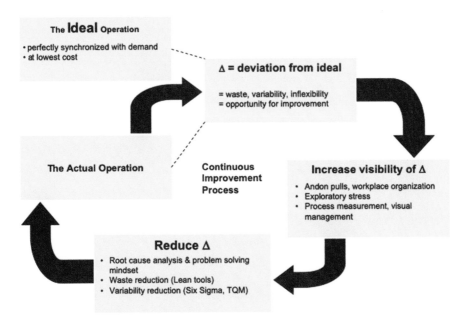

Fig. 6. A process view of continuous improvement.

4. Process improvement is a continuous journey (**Fig. 6**). The paradigm of lean operations, inspired by the Toyota Production System (further described in Anupindi and colleagues[3]), can be visualized as a continuous improvement feedback loop with the never-ending goal of waste elimination.

- Waste is any deviation between the actual process with the ideal process. This deviation is multidimensional and considers quality, time, inventory, cost, and inflexibility. Waste is an opportunity for improvement.
- Make waste visible. What is measured and visualized gets attention. The Toyota Production System uses various tools to make waste visual. The andon cord, pull control, standardized work, and constraints on buffers all serve to draw attention to problems and start the next item.
- Reduce waste with lean tools and quality tools.

DISCLOSURE

The authors have nothing to disclose.

REFERENCES

1. Takeda A, Martin N, Taylor RS, et al. Disease management interventions for heart failure. Cochrane Database Syst Rev 2019;(1):CD002752.

2. Bradley EH, Curry L, Horwitz LI, et al. Hospital strategies associated with 30-day readmission rates for patients with heart failure. Circ Cardiovasc Qual Outcomes 2013;6(4):444–50.

3. Anupindi R, Chopra S, Deshmukh SD, et al. Managing business process flows. 3rd edition. Prentice Hall;Upper Saddle River, New Jersey,2011.

4. Little JDC. A proof for the queuing formula: $L = \lambda W$. Operations Res 1961;9(3):383–7.

5. Mutharasan RK, Ahmad FS, Gurvich I, et al. Buffer or suffer: redesigning heart failure postdischarge clinic using queuing theory. Circ Cardiovasc Qual Outcomes 2018;11(7):e004351.

6. El Sayed MJ, El-Eid GR, Saliba M, et al. Improving emergency department door to doctor time and process reliability: a successful implementation of lean methodology. Medicine (Baltimore) 2015;94(42):e1679.

Identification of Patients with Heart Failure in Large Datasets

Bernard S. Kadosh, MD[a], Stuart D. Katz, MD[a], Saul Blecker, MD[b,c,d],*

KEYWORDS

• Heart failure • Machine learning • Natural language processing • Phenomapping

KEY POINTS

• Process improvement in heart failure requires identification of true heart failure cases within a large dataset.
• Identification of true cases poses unique challenges because of the syndromic nature of heart failure, variable presentations, and changing nomenclature.
• Various approaches and types of data may be used for identification of patients with heart failure, including epidemiologic, administrative, and electronic health record–based definitions.
• Machine learning and natural language processing techniques allow large-scale information processing using both structured and unstructured data, and may help define subpopulations of heart failure relevant to both clinical and research realms.

INTRODUCTION

Despite much progress in the diagnosis and treatment of chronic heart failure (HF) over the last 2 decades, the disease continues to impose a large burden on patients, caregivers, and health care systems. The lifetime risk of developing HF in a 40-year-old is 20%, with half of those patients facing mortality within 5 years of diagnosis.[1,2] The estimated annual cost of treating HF is more than $30 billion in the United States, with projections exceeding $70 billion by 2030.[1] HF is among the most common causes for hospitalizations, which account for a large proportion of this cost and morbidity for patients.[3,4] In response to this challenge, hospitals and health systems have focused their resources on improving processes such as early discharge planning, providing medications at time of discharge, scheduling close outpatient follow-up, pharmacist counseling, and postdischarge phone calls.[5,6] In addition, the Centers for Medicare and Medicaid Services began the Hospital Readmissions Reduction Program in an effort to encourage the use of evidence-based therapies shown to reduce hospitalizations.[7] The use of informatics to assist in identifying and caring for patients with HF has accelerated rapidly with a wide range of applications that have been shown to improve outcomes.[8] Hospitals can use electronic health records (EHRs) to identify patients with HF and alert specialized HF teams at the time of admission. Electronic order sets, best-practice advisories, and inpatient educational tools can be automatically summoned to promote the use of evidence-based therapies. Retrospective analysis of administrative data, and more complex analyses of data registries and EHRs, can be used for quality improvement initiatives, performance feedback, and predictive risk modeling, or to answer broad research questions about how patients with HF are characterized and treated. This article reviews the current

[a] Leon H. Charney Division of Cardiology, Department of Medicine, New York University School of Medicine, New York, NY, USA; [b] Department of Population Health, NYU School of Medicine, New York, NY, USA; [c] Department of Medicine, NYU School of Medicine, New York, NY, USA; [d] Center for Healthcare Innovation and Delivery Science, NYU Langone Health, New York, NY, USA
* Corresponding author. NYU School of Medicine, 227 East 30th St., 6th Floor, New York, NY, 10016
E-mail address: Saul.Blecker@nyulangone.org

Heart Failure Clin 16 (2020) 379–386
https://doi.org/10.1016/j.hfc.2020.05.001
1551-7136/20/© 2020 Elsevier Inc. All rights reserved.

literature outlining automated approaches to identification of patients with HF to be used for process improvement, clinical decision making, and research.

CHALLENGES IN DEFINING HEART FAILURE

The natural history of HF varies greatly among individual patients because it may present with an indolent or fulminant course, with long periods of chronic stability punctuated by unpredictable acute exacerbations. The diagnosis is challenging even for experienced clinicians because of its syndromic nature defined by a constellation of nonspecific signs and symptoms.[2,9] The lack of an HF diagnostic gold standard and the myriad of imprecise clinical terms used to describe the disease is a barrier for identification of true HF cases in administrative and epidemiologic databases.[10] Outdated terms such as diastolic HF are still used interchangeably with contemporary terms such as HF with preserved ejection fraction (HFpEF), HF with midrange ejection fraction (EF), or more general terms such as cardiomyopathy and volume overload.[11,12] Accurate identification of acute events is equally challenging, because an exacerbation may occur in the ambulatory setting; an emergency room; and in internal medicine, surgical, critical care, and cardiology hospital units with varying degrees of severity.[13,14] In addition, the relative contributions of comorbid conditions to an acute exacerbation such as renal disease, pulmonary disease, anemia, or infection is not always apparent in coding data.

Administrative databases can be powerful tools for studying large numbers of patients with HF at low cost, but their usefulness is limited by the validity of their diagnosis codes. Because these databases are not built for research purposes, validity against a gold-standard diagnosis is of particular concern. McCormick and colleagues[12] systematically reviewed studies that used administrative data and reported validation statistics for the main International Classification of Diseases (ICD) codes for HF. They found that 37% of those studies used formal diagnostic criteria (such as the Framingham, Carlson, or European Society of Cardiology criteria), which can offer a high positive predictive value but are limited by the quality of documentation. The remaining studies either used clinical chart review with unspecified diagnostic criteria or patient self-report. Chart review may be more sensitive for identification of patients with true HF but is potentially subject to bias because of interobservation variation. Objective information such as the presence of HF medications in the medication reconciliation list or

increased natriuretic peptide levels is supportive of the correct diagnosis but is subject to confounding from other disease processes.[15–17] Although HF diagnoses identified by administrative data frequently do reflect true HF cases, an estimated 25% to 30% of true HF cases are missed.[12]

APPROACHES TO COHORT IDENTIFICATION

As described earlier, large datasets pose a major challenge in the identification of predefined patient populations. In order to study an HF population, the patients must be distinguished from other cohorts that may share similar characteristics in the patient record. This article defines 2 main components in the identification of an HF cohort, whether to be used for clinical, operational, or research purposes. The first is the type of data being used, whether administrative or billing data, EHR data from the clinical record, epidemiologic data, or study data. The second component of identification is the approach to including or excluding cases in the dataset. The approach for identification of a cohort in a given dataset can range in complexity from simple searches involving 1 specific variable to advanced algorithms involving so-called big data. The identification approach can either involve automated algorithms with prespecified criteria or manual review from clinicians or other experts; the current article focuses on automated approaches for cohort identification. Nonetheless, manual chart review is frequently used as a gold standard for validation of approaches.

This article gives examples of approaches to identify patients with HF. These approaches are categorized based on datasets for which they originally were developed, including epidemiologic, claims, and EHR-based definitions (**Table 1**). These categories are fluid in relationship to the types of data; for instance, claims definitions, which are typically based on encounter diagnosis codes in an insurance data base, are frequently applied in EHR data that also have this information. In addition, these categories may not be comprehensive. For instance, this article does not discuss registry-based approaches, which are frequently based on claims or EHR-based definitions, or clinical trial–based definitions, which are beyond the scope of this article.

Regardless of the dataset being used, the approach to include or exclude cases in the cohort can also be tailored for specific uses. For instance, inclusion criteria can be developed to have a high sensitivity, which may be appropriate to estimate prevalence of disease in a given population or for

Table 1
Approaches to cohort identification in heart failure

Approach	Example	Advantages	Disadvantages
Epidemiologic	Framingham criteria	• Close to a gold standard for diagnosis	• Small-scale cohorts • Limited applicability to current clinical practice
Claims/ administrative	ICD codes	• Standardized • Data can come from multiple sources across health systems	• Lack clinical context • Numerous codes overlap similar disease states
Structured	Problem lists	• Entered by clinicians • Unambiguous • Easily searchable	• Incompletely maintained • Questionable accuracy • Snapshot in time
Unstructured	Natural language processing	• Analysis of a clinical narrative • Can contextualize information • Makes unsearchable data available for use	• Difficulty to extract accurately • Sacrifice sensitivity for specificity

implementation of a low-cost quality improvement intervention throughout a health system that can be widely disseminated (**Fig. 1**). In contrast, identification of patients with HF for enrollment in a high-cost quality improvement intervention or for recruitment into a clinical trial may be best achieved with strict criteria to achieve a high positive predictive value (PPV), even at the expense of reduced sensitivity.[15]

Epidemiologic Definitions

Several epidemiologic studies have developed approaches to define HF in their cohorts. Epidemiologic definitions of HF such as the Framingham criteria[18] and the Carlson criteria[19] rely heavily on imprecise physical examination (neck vein distension, presence of an S3, hepatomegaly) and chest radiography findings to make the diagnosis. Automated extraction of these characteristics can be challenging, so these definitions are most commonly obtained by manual chart extraction and then used as a near-gold standard to validate other approaches to cohort identification.[12] Notably, echocardiography and serum biomarkers are omitted because these criteria were developed more than 35 years ago, thus limiting their applicability to current clinical practice. In addition, physical examination findings have been shown to have questionable accuracy in the diagnosis of dyspnea.[20] Also, these definitions were based on small cohorts from an era that predates most modern prevention and treatment of cardiovascular disease and thus may not reflect the totality of contemporary HF phenotypes to be identified. Although The Atherosclerosis Risk in Communities (ARIC) study developed a more contemporary

approach to identifying HF based on detailed chart review, an attempt to develop an automated algorithm was limited in accuracy.[21]

Claims Only–Based Definition

Administrative databases contain information obtained for nonclinical reasons. They commonly consist of billing claims to insurance providers from multiple sources, such as physicians, facilities, and pharmacies. A basic approach to identify an HF cohort in these data is to search for a single instance of a diagnosis code for HF. This approach relies on the assumption that an accurate diagnosis has been made and coded accordingly.

McCormick and colleagues[12] conducted a systematic review of studies through 2009 that validated claims-based definitions for HF. The PPV was at least 87% in most studies, whereas the pooled sensitivity was 75%. More recently, a study of the Danish National Patient Register using ICD-10 codes found that a primary HF diagnosis had a PPV of 88% for HF cases deemed probable or definite based on chart review.[22] Li and colleagues[23] examined ICD-9 codes related to systolic HF and combined systolic and diastolic HF to identify patients with HF with reduced EF (HFrEF). The presence of 1 of these codes had a sensitivity of 97.1% and PPV of 76.7% for systolic dysfunction, compared with documented EF less than 45%. Huang and colleagues[24] found that the ICD-9 code for HF alone had a sensitivity of 97.5% for identifying acute decompensated HF admissions in the Veterans' Affairs (VA) system. When combined with codes such as acute edema of lung unspecified, sensitivity improved to 99.2%. A Canadian study of ICD-10 codes in the emergency

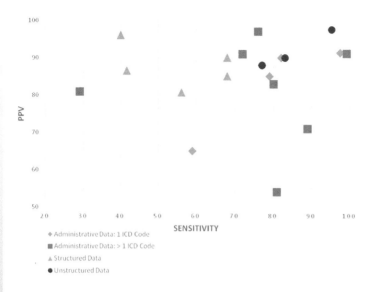

Fig. 1. Positive predictive value and sensitivity for HF cohort identification from selection of prior studies, categorized by type of data. Compilation of reported sensitivities and positive predictive values (PPV) for automated identification of HF cohorts using administrative,[24,28] structured,[15,21,38] and unstructured data[38,40] validated either by chart review or epidemiologic criteria. There is frequently a tradeoff between sensitivity and PPV, and the chosen approach may depend on the goal of the cohort identification. For instance, high-sensitivity and low-PPV definitions may be appropriate for screening or low-cost process improvement interventions, whereas lower-sensitivity and high-PPV definitions may be more appropriate for resource-intensive interventions or recruitment for clinical trials.

department setting had only modest sensitivity (76.1%) but a high PPV (93.3%) for identification of HF cases compared with the Carlson criteria.[25] Other studies have concluded that the use of ICD-9 codes alone is not sufficient to accurately phenotype patients across multiple disease states.[26,27] An analysis of 25 studies that used ICD codes to define patients with HF revealed wide variability in reported sensitivity (29% to 89%), and PPV (12% to 100%).[28]

Electronic Health Record–Based Definitions

Because most contemporary clinical care and documentation is funneled through the EHR, the EHR has become a primary target for identifying cohorts of patients with HF. Most EHRs contain administrative or encounter data using for billing, such that simple claims-based definitions can be applied to EHR data, as well as both structured clinical data and unstructured information in the form of clinical narratives written by providers. Extraction of meaningful and useable information from these 2 types of data poses unique challenges.

Structured electronic health record data
Structured data may include problem lists, laboratory values, and medications. These data are easily searchable and well suited for large-scale analysis across multiple health systems and data networks. For example, the Patient Centered Outcomes Research Network (PCORnet) is a nationwide platform for observational studies and contains only structured data elements but allows for large-scale recruitment into clinical trials.[29]

Various algorithms have been used to analyze a combination of claims and other structured data in order to accurately phenotype HF cohorts.[30–33] Tison and colleagues[15] evaluated the performance of a simple algorithm (the presence of ≥1 HF diagnostic code in the EHR) against more increasingly complicated algorithms that incorporated multiple inpatient and outpatient diagnostic codes, HF medications, and increased N-terminal pro–brain natriuretic peptide level. The simplest algorithms offered the highest sensitivity, whereas the most complicated had the highest PPV for true HF cases at the expense of sensitivity.

However, structured data are not always reliable in terms of accurately reflecting patient phenotypes. Problem lists are problems in and of themselves for providers, who have varying attitudes about what should or should not be included, how to reflect changes in disease states over time, and who should be responsible for managing and maintaining the list.[34] Studies of problem lists in the VA system as well as EHRs in the United Kingdom and Australia have found completeness rates ranging from 60.2% to 99.4%.[35,36]

Unstructured electronic health record data
Unstructured data in the EHR consist of free text documentation, including provider notes, discharge summaries, and results from diagnostic procedures such as echocardiograms and radiology reports. Although this information contains complex clinical narratives that can ideally be extracted to define a clinical picture, the presence of nonstandardized abbreviations, grammatical errors, misspelled words, colloquialisms, and

regional or institution-specific terms complicates the search strategy. Techniques such as natural language processing (NLP) have been used to leverage massive amounts of heterogeneous data of this type. The Congestive Heart Failure Information Extraction Framework (CHIEF), developed by the VA, is an NLP application system used to identify HF cohorts in order to assess whether patients with HF are being prescribed guideline-directed medical therapy appropriately.[37] CHIEF was applied to the EHR using modules to process clinical text; analyze sentences and syntax; and extract mentions of EF, mentions of medications, and quantitative variables. Performance measures were assessed by applying a set of rules to the extracted data. Compared with a human-annotated reference standard, the NLP system was able to accurately extract relevant mentions of medications and EF with at least 96% sensitivity and 88% PPV.

Increasingly, machine learning approaches to define HF cohorts are being evaluated using both structured and unstructured data in commercial EHRs as well. Blecker and colleagues[38] compared 5 algorithms of increasing complexity. The first 3 used the problem list, medications, brain natriuretic peptide levels, and 30 other clinically relevant structured data. The last 2 algorithms used machine learning with unstructured notes, and machine learning with structured and unstructured elements. Machine learning performed with the highest accuracy, showing an area under the receiver operating curve (AUC) of 0.97 for identification of HF cases. Follow-up work in the early identification of patients with acutely decompensated HF showed an AUC of 0.99 for machine learning with structured and unstructured elements.[39] Evans and colleagues[40] reported an NLP system that identified patients with HF admitted to the hospital and assigned a 30-day readmission risk score and a 30-day mortality risk score based on prespecified criteria. The use of this system resulted in a reduction in 30-day mortality and more patients discharged to home care rather than to a facility. This example shows the potential for informatics to directly affect patient outcomes by first identifying vulnerable populations that otherwise would not receive special attention. Real-time use of informatics in the inpatient setting has been used to alert specialized teams to the presence of patients with HF, provide reminders to incorporate evidence-based therapies, and as a quality improvement instrument to assess provider-level and hospital-level performance.[5,8]

Although NLP and machine learning techniques have demonstrable patient care applications, the implications for epidemiologic research are equally impressive. The Electronic Medical Records and Genomics (eMERGE) Network developed an EHR algorithm using NLP with structured and unstructured data to phenotype patients with HF with a PPV of greater than 95%.[41]

PHENOMAPPING SUBGROUP IDENTIFICATION

Recently, some approaches to identify patients with HF have moved beyond simple identification of the disease to development of clustering algorithms that define subgroups of similar patients with HF. This approach has most commonly been used by classifying patients as HFrEF versus HFpEF, given the difference in treatment recommendations between the 2 groups. For instance, the eMERGE Network has worked to extract the EF from radiology reports, allowing their algorithm to differentiate HFrEF from HFpEF phenotypes.[41]

Beyond this, machine learning algorithms can combine structured and unstructured elements to cluster similar patients using large quantities of data. Beyond the identification of true HF cases in the EHR, this capability has opened the possibility of redefining the disease itself. HFpEF remains a vexing disease entity for clinicians and clinical trialists, who have yet to characterize its heterogeneity. Using a machine learning approach, Shah and colleagues[42] clustered 397 patients with HFpEF into 3 distinct groups that differed in age, comorbidities, hemodynamics, and clinical outcomes including death and HF hospitalizations. In pursuit of a more nuanced classification of HF beyond EF, another study using a large cohort of 44,886 patients enrolled in the Swedish Heart Registry performed a cluster analysis of patients with HF irrespective of left ventricular function.[43] It identified 4 distinct clinically recognizable HF phenotypes, each with separate 1-year survival curves and differences in benefit from common HF therapies. Although these data were retrospective, the implication is a potential pathway for reclassifying the disease, individualizing care, and refinement in the design of clinical trials toward the development of novel therapies.

FUTURE DIRECTIONS

HF continues to be a pressing public health issue that is growing in complexity as the population ages. The advent of EHRs and availability of large databases have afforded unprecedented opportunities for epidemiologic research and improvement of quality care delivery. To that end, efforts should be made toward standardizing the terminology used for HF across clinical and research institutions commensurate with the definitions used in clinical practice guidelines. Coding for HF disease states should be simplified to reflect commonly used clinical language in order to decrease heterogeneity across databases. In addition, cross-compatibility among various EHRs with the ubiquitous availability of clinically structured data elements (such as EF) would greatly broaden the utility of these systems and increase efficiency for both clinicians and researchers.[44]

As machine learning approaches become more sophisticated, incorporating larger datasets, algorithms could be developed to estimate the probability of clinical outcomes. Risk factors and genomic data have been used to predict outcomes in breast, brain, and ovarian cancers.[45–47] Similarly, predictive modeling may identify patients who are more likely to have sudden cardiac death, or who may respond to one medication rather than another. There remains a great need to identify patients with stage D HF for early consideration of advanced therapies before clinical deterioration puts them at higher risk of morbidity and mortality. In addition, the use of phenomapping techniques opens the door to potentially redefine subsets of HF populations, improve the current understanding of HF as a clinical syndrome, and direct research efforts toward novel therapeutic approaches.

DISCLOSURE

The authors have nothing to disclose.

REFERENCES

1. Benjamin EJ, Virani SS, Callaway CW, et al. American Heart Association Council on Epidemiology and Prevention Statistics Committee and Stroke Statistics Subcommittee. Heart disease and stroke statistics-2018 update: a report from the American Heart Association. Circulation 2018;137(12): e67–492.
2. Yancy CW, Jessup M, Bozkurt B, et al. 2017 ACC/AHA/HFSA focused update of the 2013 ACCF/AHA guideline for the management of heart failure: a report of the American College of Cardiology/American Heart Association Task Force on clinical practice guidelines and the Heart Failure Society of America. J Am Coll Cardiol 2017;70(6):776–803.
3. Blecker S, Paul M, Taksler G, et al. Heart failure-associated hospitalizations in the United States. J Am Coll Cardiol 2013;61(12):1259–67.
4. Jencks SF, Williams MV, Coleman EA. Rehospitalizations among patients in the Medicare fee-for-service program. N Engl J Med 2009;360(14):1418–28.
5. Kociol RD, Peterson ED, Hammill BG, et al. National survey of hospital strategies to reduce heart failure readmissions: findings from the Get With the Guidelines-Heart Failure registry. Circ Heart Fail 2012;5(6):680–7.
6. Vasilevskis EE, Kripalani S, Ong MK, et al. Variability in implementation of interventions aimed at reducing readmissions among patients with heart failure: a survey of teaching hospitals. Acad Med 2016; 91(4):522–9.
7. Centers for Medicare & Medicaid Services. Hospital readmissions reduction program. Available at: https://www.cms.gov/Medicare/Medicare-Fee-for-Service-Payment/AcuteInpatientPPS/Readmissions-Reduction-Program. Accessed November 18, 2019.
8. Banerjee D, Thompson C, Bingham A, et al. An electronic medical record report improves identification of hospitalized patients with heart failure. J Card Fail 2015;22(5):402–5.
9. Ponikowski P, Voors AA, Anker SD, et al, ESC Scientific Document Group. 2016 ESC Guidelines for the diagnosis and treatment of acute and chronic heart failure: The Task Force for the diagnosis and treatment of acute and chronic heart failure of the European Society of Cardiology (ESC)Developed with the special contribution of the Heart Failure Association (HFA) of the ESC. Eur Heart J 2016;37(27): 2129–200.
10. Cainzos-Achirica M, Rebordosa C, Vela E, et al. Challenges of evaluating chronic heart failure and acute heart failure events in research studies using large health care databases. Am Heart J 2018;202: 76–83.
11. Packer M. Heart failure with a mid-range ejection fraction: a disorder that a psychiatrist would love. JACC Heart Fail 2017;5(11):805–7.
12. McCormick N, Lacaille D, Bhole V, et al. Validity of heart failure diagnoses in administrative databases: a systematic review and meta-analysis. PLoS One 2014;9(8):e104519.
13. Komajda M. Current challenges in the management of heart failure. Circ J 2015;79(5):948–53.
14. Metra M, Cotter G, El-Khorazaty J, et al. Acute heart failure in the elderly: differences in clinical characteristics, outcomes, and prognostic factors in the VERITAS Study. J Card Fail 2015;21(3):179–88.
15. Tison GH, Chamberlain AM, Pletcher MJ, et al. Identifying heart failure using EMR-based algorithms. Int J Med Inform 2018;120:1–7.
16. Rosenman M, He J, Martin J, et al. Database queries for hospitalizations for acute congestive heart failure: flexible methods and validation based on set theory. J Am Med Inform Assoc 2014;21(2):345–52.
17. Januzzi JL, van Kimmenade R, Lainchbury J, et al. NT-proBNP testing for diagnosis and short-term prognosis in acute destabilized heart failure: an international pooled analysis of 1256 patients: the

International Collaborative of NT-proBNP Study. Eur Heart J 2006;27(3):330–7.

18. McKee PA, Castelli WP, McNamara PM, et al. The natural history of congestive heart failure: the Framingham study. N Engl J Med 1971;285(26):1441–6.

19. Carlson KJ, Lee DC, Goroll AH, et al. An analysis of physicians' reasons for prescribing long-term digitalis therapy in outpatients. J Chronic Dis 1985; 38(9):733–9.

20. Marantz PR, Kaplan MC, Alderman MH. Clinical diagnosis of congestive heart failure in patients with acute dyspnea. Chest 1990;97(4):776–81.

21. Loehr LR, Agarwal SK, Baggett C, et al. Classification of acute decompensated heart failure: an automated algorithm compared with a physician reviewer panel: the Atherosclerosis Risk in Communities study. Circ Heart Fail 2013;6(4):719–26.

22. Delekta J, Hansen SM, AlZuhairi KS, et al. The validity of the diagnosis of heart failure (I50.0-I50.9) in the Danish National Patient Register. Dan Med J 2018; 65(4) [pii:A5470].

23. Li Q, Glynn RJ, Dreyer NA, et al. Validity of claims-based definitions of left ventricular systolic dysfunction in Medicare patients. Pharmacoepidemiol Drug Saf 2011;20(7):700–8.

24. Huang H, Turner M, Raju S, et al. Identification of acute decompensated heart failure hospitalizations using administrative data. Am J Cardiol 2017; 119(11):1791–6.

25. Frolova N, Bakal JA, McAlister FA, et al. Assessing the use of international classification of diseases-10th revision codes from the emergency department for the identification of acute heart failure. JACC Heart Fail 2015;3(5):386–91.

26. Shivade C, Raghavan P, Fosler-Lussier E, et al. A review of approaches to identifying patient phenotype cohorts using electronic health records. J Am Med Inform Assoc 2014;21(2):221–30.

27. Birman-Deych E, Waterman AD, Yan Y, et al. Accuracy of ICD-9-CM codes for identifying cardiovascular and stroke risk factors. Med Care 2005;43(5): 480–5.

28. Quach S, Blais C, Quan H. Administrative data have high variation in validity for recording heart failure. Can J Cardiol 2010;26(8):306–12.

29. Fleurence RL, Curtis LH, Califf RM, et al. Launching PCORnet, a national patient-centered clinical research network. J Am Med Inform Assoc 2014; 21(4):578–82.

30. Saczynski JS, Andrade SE, Harrold LR, et al. A systematic review of validated methods for identifying heart failure using administrative data. Pharmacoepidemiol Drug Saf 2012;21(Suppl 1):129–40.

31. Wright A, Pang J, Feblowitz JC, et al. A method and knowledge base for automated inference of patient problems from structured data in an electronic medical record. J Am Med Inform Assoc 2011; 18(6):859–67.

32. Newton KM, Peissig PL, Kho AN, et al. Validation of electronic medical record-based phenotyping algorithms: results and lessons learned from the eMERGE network. J Am Med Inform Assoc 2013; 20(e1):e147–54.

33. Pathak J, Kho AN, Denny JC. Electronic health records-driven phenotyping: challenges, recent advances, and perspectives. J Am Med Inform Assoc 2013;20(e2):e206–11.

34. Holmes C, Brown M, Hilaire DS, et al. Healthcare provider attitudes towards the problem list in an electronic health record: a mixed-methods qualitative study. BMC Med Inform Decis Mak 2012;12:127.

35. Szeto HC, Coleman RK, Gholami P, et al. Accuracy of computerized outpatient diagnoses in a Veterans Affairs general medicine clinic. Am J Manag Care 2002;8(1):37–43.

36. Wright A, McCoy AB, Hickman TT, et al. Problem list completeness in electronic health records: A multi-site study and assessment of success factors. Int J Med Inform 2015;84(10):784–90.

37. Garvin JH, Kim Y, Gobbel GT, et al. Automating quality measures for heart failure using natural language processing: a descriptive study in the department of veterans affairs. JMIR Med Inform 2018;6(1):e5.

38. Blecker S, Katz SD, Horwitz LI, et al. Comparison of approaches for heart failure case identification from electronic health record data. JAMA Cardiol 2016; 1(9):1014–20.

39. Blecker S, Sontag D, Horwitz LI, et al. Early identification of patients with acute decompensated heart failure. J Card Fail 2018;24(6):357–62.

40. Evans RS, Benuzillo J, Horne BD, et al. Automated identification and predictive tools to help identify high-risk heart failure patients: pilot evaluation. J Am Med Inform Assoc 2016;23(5):872–8.

41. Bielinski SJ, Pathak J, Carrell DS, et al. A robust e-epidemiology tool in phenotyping heart failure with differentiation for preserved and reduced ejection fraction: the electronic medical records and genomics (eMERGE) Network. J Cardiovasc Transl Res 2015;8(8):475–83.

42. Shah SJ, Katz DH, Selvaraj S, et al. Phenomapping for novel classification of heart failure with preserved ejection fraction. Circulation 2015;131(3):269–79.

43. Ahmad T, Lund LH, Rao P, et al. Machine learning methods improve prognostication, identify clinically distinct phenotypes, and detect heterogeneity in response to therapy in a large cohort of heart failure patients. J Am Heart Assoc 2018;7(8) [pii:e008081].

44. Conway M, Berg RL, Carrell D, et al. Analyzing the heterogeneity and complexity of Electronic Health Record oriented phenotyping algorithms. AMIA Annu Symp Proc 2011;2011:274–83.

45. Singleton KW, Hsu W, Bui AA. Comparing predictive models of glioblastoma multiforme built using multi-institutional and local data sources. AMIA Annu Symp Proc 2012;2012:1385–92.

46. Tatari F, Akbarzadeh-T MR, Sabahi A. Fuzzy-probabilistic multi agent system for breast cancer risk assessment and insurance premium assignment. J Biomed Inform 2012;45(6):1021–34.

47. Kim D, Shin H, Song YS, et al. Synergistic effect of different levels of genomic data for cancer clinical outcome prediction. J Biomed Inform 2012;45(6): 1191–8.

Predicting High-Risk Patients and High-Risk Outcomes in Heart Failure

Ramsey M. Wehbe, MD[a], Sadiya S. Khan, MD, MSc[a,b], Sanjiv J. Shah, MD[a], Faraz S. Ahmad, MD, MS[a,b,c],*

KEYWORDS

- Heart failure - Prognosis - Risk factors - Risk models - Risk scores - Artificial intelligence
- Machine learning - Deep learning

KEY POINTS

- Identifying patients with heart failure who are at high risk for poor outcomes is important for patient care, resource allocation and process improvement.
- Several risk models exist to identify high-risk patients with heart failure, based on traditional statistical risk modeling methodology.
- Risk models for heart failure are infrequently used in practice because of their modest performance outside validation cohorts, lack of evidence to support that risk modeling in heart failure improves outcomes, and barriers to implementation.
- Machine learning may offer an alternative solution for a precision medicine approach to personalized risk prediction in patients with heart failure, but has its own limitations.
- The future of risk prediction in heart failure will likely involve more sophisticated risk modeling, incorporating diverse data sources not typically included in existing risk scores.

Prediction is very difficult...especially if it's about the future.

—Niels Bohr

INTRODUCTION

More than 6.5 million Americans are now living with heart failure (HF) and the prevalence continues to increase.[1] Despite substantial advances in medical therapy, many patients progress to end-stage disease with a 5-year absolute mortality of approximately 50%.[2] Moreover, HF is a significant burden on the United States health care system, accounting for ~800,000 hospitalizations in 2016 and projected to cost $69.7 billion annually by the year 2030.[1,3]

Identifying high-risk patients with HF is therefore an important, but challenging, pursuit for clinicians and health care systems alike. Prognosis of individual patients with HF is highly variable in contemporary cohorts, and the risk of serious clinical outcomes such as mortality and hospitalization for HF can differ more than 20-fold.[4,5] Predicting adverse outcomes in patients with HF could theoretically help direct resources to patients at the highest levels of risk who might benefit

---

[a] Division of Cardiology, Department of Medicine, Northwestern University Feinberg School of Medicine, 676 North St. Clair Street, Suite 600, Chicago, IL 60611, USA; [b] Department of Preventive Medicine, Northwestern University Feinberg School of Medicine, 680 N Lake Shore Drive, Suite 1400, Chicago, IL 60611, USA; [c] Center for Health Information Partnerships, Institute for Public Health and Medicine, Northwestern University Feinberg School of Medicine, 625 N Michigan Avenue, 15th Floor, Chicago, IL 60611, USA

* Corresponding author. 676 North Saint Clair Street, Suite 600, Chicago, IL 60611.

E-mail address: faraz.ahmad@northwestern.edu

Twitter: @ramseywehbemd (R.M.W.); @HeartDocSadiya (S.S.K.); @HFpEF (S.J.S.); @FarazA_MD (F.S.A.)

Heart Failure Clin 16 (2020) 387–407
https://doi.org/10.1016/j.hfc.2020.05.002
1551-7136/20/© 2020 Elsevier Inc. All rights reserved.

the most from earlier and more intensive monitoring and treatment (eg, targeted medications, cardiac devices, home monitoring systems, and social services), while avoiding unnecessary interventions and costs for patients at low risk.[6–9] Ideally, this would translate into improved outcomes and cost-efficiency in providing care for patients with HF. Given the importance of risk prediction for process improvement in HF, this article reviews the available evidence on prognostic variables and the current state of risk prediction for patients with HF. In addition, it discusses the limitations of traditional risk modeling and provides a glimpse into the future of risk prediction in HF.

ESTABLISHED RISK FACTORS FOR POOR OUTCOMES IN PATIENTS WITH HEART FAILURE

Several demographic and clinical variables have been explored as markers of increased risk for adverse outcomes in HF populations. Risk factors can vary substantially based on the outcome of interest or the population under study. Although a discussion of all of these risk factors is beyond the scope of this article, some of the prognostic features that have been consistently found to be

significant drivers of clinically important outcomes, including mortality, hospitalization, and health-related quality of life (HRQOL) measures, are summarized in **Box 1**. Risk factors are derived from various domains, including demographics, clinical characteristics, functional status and HF grade (**Table 1**), comorbidities, vital signs, laboratory tests, imaging, hemodynamics, exercise capacity, medication and device therapy adherence, and social determinants of health.

MULTIVARIABLE RISK MODELS FOR PATIENTS WITH HEART FAILURE

Considerable effort has been devoted to developing multivariable risk scores to help summarize and simplify risk assessment so that it can be performed in real time in a clinical setting or embedded into systems of care. To date, hundreds of multivariable risk scores for predicting outcomes in HF populations have been developed. Most of these risk models have been derived from multivariable statistical modeling, such as logistic regression (LR) and Cox proportional hazards analysis. Some of these scores are derived directly from parameter estimates of regression models and involve complex

---

Box 1
Established risk factors for poor prognosis in patients with heart failure

Demographics[14,15,76–80]: age, sex, race/ethnicity

Systolic and diastolic dysfunction[41–45,81]

HF cause[82,83] (eg, ischemic vs nonischemic)

Functional class,[84–86] HF stage,[87] INTERMACS (Interagency Registry for Mechanically Assisted Circulatory Support) profile[88]

Body Mass Index[89]: cardiac cachexia and the obesity paradox

Comorbidities[2,25,90–94]: diabetes, renal dysfunction, liver disease, chronic obstructive pulmonary disease, anemia, depression

Vital signs[95–99]: hypotension, heart rate (HR), HR variability

Electrophysiologic risk factors[100–104]: arrhythmias (atrial fibrillation, ventricular tachycardia/ ventricular fibrillation), QRS prolongation

Laboratory values[105–110]: sodium, biomarkers (natriuretic peptides, troponin, novel biomarkers [soluble ST2, galectin-3, growth differentiation factor-15])

Imaging[111–116]: chamber enlargement, right ventricular dysfunction, strain imaging, delayed gadolinium enhancement

Hemodynamics[117–123]: increased filling pressures, pulmonary hypertension, cardiac index, exercise hemodynamics

Exercise capacity[124–126]: peak oxygen uptake (Vo_2), 6-minute walk test

Prior hospitalization for HF[127–129]

Underuse of guideline-directed medical therapies[130–132]

Social determinants of health[133–136]

Table 1
American College of Cardiology Foundation/American Heart Association heart failure stage, New York Heart Association functional class, and Interagency Registry for Mechanically Assisted Circulatory Support profiles[84,87,88]

ACCF/AHA Stages	NYHA Class	INTERMACS Profile
(A) At risk for HF, but no structural heart disease	—	—
(B) Structural heart disease, but no symptoms or limitations	(I) Asymptomatic, no physical limitations	—
(C) Structural heart disease with current or prior HF symptoms	(II) Symptomatic with moderate exertion, slight limitation in activity	—
	(III) Symptomatic with minimal exertion, marked limitation in activity	(7) Advanced NYHA III (6) Exertion limited
(D) End-stage disease, refractory HF requiring specialized interventions	(IV) Symptomatic at rest, not capable of exertion	(5) Exertion intolerant (4) Resting symptoms (3) Inotrope dependent, but stable (2) Progressive decline (1) Critical cardiogenic shock

Abbreviations: ACCF, American College of Cardiology Foundation; AHA, American Heart Association; INTERMACS, Interagency Registry for Mechanically Assisted Circulatory Support; NYHA, New York Heart Association.

calculations, whereas others have been translated into nomograms with integer scores given to different covariates based on their relative contribution to the overall risk.

Because the risk factors that contribute to adverse outcomes can vary substantially based on the HF population (eg, HF with reduced ejection fraction [HFrEF] vs HF with preserved ejection fraction [HFpEF]) or health care delivery setting (eg, inpatient vs outpatient), risk models have been developed for use in specific cohorts, including those with chronic ambulatory HF, hospitalized HF (HHF), and HFpEF specifically. The most popular and well-validated clinical multivariable risk scores for HF are summarized in **Table 2**, and key features of these risk models are discussed in more detail later. Notably, many of the risk factors discussed previously are shared by several of these multivariable risk models.

The Transparent Reporting of a Multivariable Prediction Model for Individual Prognosis or Diagnosis (TRIPOD) statement was a consortium document released in 2015 that was intended to improve the reporting of research surrounding the development and validation of risk scores.[10,11] The characteristics of model derivation and validation cohorts, outcome of interest, statistical analysis methods, handling of missing data, and measures of performance (eg, discrimination and

calibration) of the model should be clearly defined. Model discrimination, or the ability of a model to distinguish between cases and noncases, is often measured by the concordance statistic (c-statistic) which is equal to the area under the receiver operator statistic curve (AUC) for an LR model. By convention, an AUC less than 0.70 indicates inadequate discrimination for clinical use, whereas an AUC of 0.7 to 0.8 is considered acceptable and an AUC greater than 0.8 is considered excellent.[12] Model calibration refers to a model's ability to accurately predict absolute risk. This ability is often reported graphically, but there are also several statistical tests of overall calibration that are available.[13] When available, this article comments on the features discussed earlier; however, frequently these are not reported for existing HF risk models.

Chronic Ambulatory Heart Failure

Numerous risk models have been developed to predict clinical outcomes in cohorts of ambulatory patients with HF.[14–18] Most of these models have focused on all-cause mortality as the outcome of interest and have examined more intermediate-term to long-term outcomes given that short-term event rates are typically low in ambulatory populations. Notably, most of the risk models for patients with chronic HF share a core set of common risk factors, including age, sex, New York

Table 2
Popular clinical multivariable risk prediction models for patients with heart failure

Risk Model	Multivariate Predictors	Outcomes
Chronic HF		
Seattle Heart Failure Model[19] (2006)	Age, sex, LVEF, NYHA class, weight, SBP, laboratory tests (Hgb, Lymphs, UA, Chol, Na), wide QRS/LBBB, medications (including GDMT, allopurinol, statins, diuretics), devices (ICD/CRT/PPM)	1-y, 2, and 5-y mortality
CHARM Risk Score[25] (2006)	Age, sex, LVEF, NYHA class, BMI, DM, AF, MR, MI, prior HF hosp, HF duration, current smoker, DBP, HR, dependent edema, pulmonary crackles, dyspnea, pulmonary edema, cardiomegaly, ARB	All-cause mortality; CV death or HF hosp
CORONA Risk Score[26] (2009)	Age, sex, LVEF, NYHA class, BMI, DM, MI, CABG, AF, claudication, HR, NT-proBNP, Cr, ApoA-1	CV death, nonfatal MI, or stroke
GISSI-HF Model[27] (2013)	Age, sex, LVEF, NYHA class, BMI, DM, COPD, AS, SBP, Laboratory tests (eGFR, Hgb, UA, NT-proBNP, hs-CTnT)	All-cause mortality
MAGGIC Risk Score[22] (2013)	Age, sex, LVEF, NYHA class, BMI, DM, COPD, recent diagnosis, smoking status, SBP, Cr, medications (β-blockers, ACEi/ARB)	1-y and 3-y all-cause mortality
PARADIGM Risk Score[28] (2020)	Age, sex, race, LVEF, NYHA class, BMI, DM, region, HF duration, HF hosp, MI, valve dz, BBB, PCI, PAD, SBP, Bili, AST, UA, Alb, K, Cl, Hgb, LDL, Trig, BUN, WBCs, NT-proBNP, β-blocker, ARNI	CV death or HF hosp; CV death; all-cause death
Hosp HF		
EFFECT Model[137] (2003)	Age, COPD, cirrhosis, cancer, dementia, cerebrovascular dz, SBP, RR, Na, BUN, Hgb	30-d and 1-y mortality
OPTIME-CHF Model[9] (2004)	Age, NYHA class, SBP, BUN, Na Prior HF hosp, SBP, BUN, h/o PCI	60-d mortality 60-d readmission
ADHERE CART Model[4] (2005)	SBP, BUN, Cr	In-hospital mortality
OPTIMIZE-HF Nomogram[37,38] (2008)	Age, LVEF, HF primary diagnosis, HR, SBP, Na, Cr Age, weight, SBP, Na, Cr, liver dz, depression, reactive airway dz	In-hospital mortality 60-d mortality or readmission
GWTG-HF Score[5] (2010)	Age, race, COPD, SBP, HR, Na, BUN	In-hospital mortality

(continued on next page)

Table 2
(continued)

Risk Model	Multivariate Predictors	Outcomes
ESCAPE Risk Score[6] (2010)	Age, CPR/mechanical ventilation, Na, BNP, BUN, diuretic, β-blocker, 6MWT	6-mo mortality
Refractory HF Risk Score[58] (2011)	Age, DM, stroke, arrhythmia, Na, BNP, BUN, β-blocker, KCCQ score	Unfavorable QOL or death at 6 mo
PROTECT HF Postdischarge Model[39] (2014)	Age, SBP, Na, Cr, BUN, albumin, prior HF hosp, peripheral edema	30/180-d mortality, all-cause hosp, and/or CV hosp
BIOSTAT-CHF Model[40] (2017)	Age, BUN, NT-proBNP, Hgb, β-blocker Age, prior HF hosp, edema, SBP, eGFR	All-cause mortality HF hosp
HFpEF		
I-PRESERVE Score[45] (2011)	Age, LVEF, ischemic cause, prior HF hosp, QOL, DM, MI, COPD/asthma, HR, eGFR, neutrophils, NT-proBNP	All-cause mortality or CV hosp, all-cause mortality, HF hosp, or mortality
ARIC Score[46] (2017)	Modified EFFECT score + race, BMI, AF, HR, hypoxia, natriuretic peptides	28-d and 1-y mortality

Abbreviations: 6MWT, 6-minute walk test; AF, atrial fibrillation; BUN, blood urea nitrogen; CART, classification and regression tree; Chol, cholesterol; COPD, chronic obstructive pulmonary disease; Cr, creatinine; CRT, cardiac resynchronization therapy; CV, cardiovascular; DBP, diastolic blood pressure; DM, diabetes mellitus; GDMT, guideline-directed medical therapy; Hgb, hemoglobin; Hosp, hospitalization; ICD, implantable cardioverter-defibrillator; KCCQ, Kansas City Cardiomyopathy Questionnaire; LBBB, left bundle branch block; LVEF, left ventricular ejection fraction; Lymphs, lymphocytes; Meds, medications; NT-proBNP, N-terminal pro–brain natriuretic peptide; PPM, permanent pacemaker; SBP, systolic blood pressure; UA, uric acid; WBC, white blood cells.

Heart Association (NYHA) class, body mass index (BMI), diabetes mellitus, systolic blood pressure (SBP), and indices of renal function.

Perhaps the most popular and thoroughly validated risk model in the chronic ambulatory HF population is the Seattle Heart Failure Model (SHFM).[19] The SHFM was derived from a clinical trial cohort (Prospective Randomized Amlodipine Survival Evaluation-1 (PRAISE-1) trial)[20] of 1125 patients with HFrEF (≤30%) and NYHA class III or IV symptoms. The components of the risk model were selected via a multivariable stepwise Cox proportional hazards model designed to predict 1-year, 2-year, and 3-year mortality. The SHFM was externally validated in 5 separate clinical trial cohorts totaling 9942 patients from varying populations (HFrEF only, mixed HFrEF/HFpEF, varying functional status and age) with discriminative performance ranging from 0.682 to 0.810 for predicting 1-year mortality and excellent calibration (correlation coefficient ≥0.97 between predicted and actual survival for all validation cohorts). The model incorporates 14 continuous variables and 10 categorical variables, including demographics, laboratory tests, electrocardiogram findings, medications, and device therapy. The investigators created an interactive online calculator to facilitate clinical use (https://depts.washington.edu/shfm). Because the SHFM was derived from an HF clinical trial cohort almost 30 years ago, before the widespread use of contemporary guideline-directed medical therapy (GDMT), performance in more modern cohorts, especially at the individual level, has been highly variable and modest at best.[21] Interestingly, the SHFM seems to overestimate survival in contemporary HF cohorts, likely explained by effect sizes for individual medications and implantable cardioverter defibrillator or cardiac resynchronization therapy use being imputed from results of large randomized clinical trials available at the time.[17,18] Often, these trials were conducted in a cohort that largely was not on a background of contemporary GDMT, thus likely overestimating individual effect sizes (and consequently overall additive benefit) of these therapies.

More recently, the Meta-Analysis Global Group in Chronic Heart Failure (MAGGIC) developed a

HF risk score using data on 39,372 patients from 30 cohort studies in an attempt to improve the ability to generalize.[22] The derivation cohorts included patients with HFrEF and HFpEF from both randomized clinical trials and observational studies. Individual components of the model were determined using Poisson regression models with forward stepwise variable selection for the outcome of mortality. Missing data were handled via multiple imputation analysis, a more robust method to handle missing variables than the methods used in most other risk prediction model derivation strategies. A total of 13 independent predictors were included in the final model, and separate models were derived for patients with HFpEF and HFrEF. Much like the SHFM, the investigators provide an online calculator for computing the MAGGIC risk score at the point of care (www.heartfailurerisk.org). Subsequently, the MAGGIC score has been validated in 51,043 patients from a large HF registry cohort (AUC = 0.741 for predicting 3-year mortality)[23] and specifically in 407 patients with HFpEF from a single-institution real-world cohort (AUC = 0.74 for predicting mortality).[24] In general, calibration plots in these validation cohorts showed slight underestimation of risk of mortality in high-risk patients and overestimation of risk of mortality in low-risk patients, with better calibration for predicting risk of hospitalization events than the SHFM.

Other notable models that have been developed for predicting outcomes in chronic ambulatory HF include the Candesartan in Heart Failure Assessment of Reduction in Mortality and Morbidity (CHARM),[25] Controlled Rosuvastatin Multinational Trial in Heart Failure (CORONA),[26] and Gruppo Italiano per lo Studio della Streptochinasi nell'Infarto Miocardico-Heart Failure (GISSI-HF)[27] risk models, all of which were derived from clinical trial cohorts. Models derived in clinical trial cohorts are limited by nonrepresentative patient populations because of significant under-recruitment of women and minorities as well as strict inclusion/exclusion criteria and thus have limited ability to generalize.

Recently, several popular risk scores for chronic ambulatory patients with HF were directly compared in a large contemporary European HF registry of more than 6000 patients.[18] The MAGGIC score had the best overall discriminatory power for estimating 1-year mortality (AUC 0.743), but all scores were only modest predictors (AUC 0.714–0.743). Moreover, calibration was poor across all risk scores, with the MAGGIC, CHARM, and GISSI-HF scores underestimating survival (given they were derived in patients with low background use of contemporary GDMT) and SHFM overestimating survival as explained previously.

Importantly, all of these risk scores were developed before the advent of angiotensin-receptor neprilysin inhibitors (ARNIs). A novel risk score was recently published using data from 8399 patients in the Prospective Comparison of ARNI with ACEI to Determine Impact on Global Mortality and Morbidity in Heart Failure (PARADIGM-HF) trial of sacubitril-valsartan.[28] Three separate models were derived for outcomes of cardiovascular death, all-cause mortality, and the composite of cardiovascular death or HF hospitalization (AUCs of 0.73, 0.71, and 0.74 at 1 year, respectively). The models were also validated using data from ~7000 patients in the Aliskiren Trial to Minimize Outcomes in Patients with Heart Failure (ATMOSPHERE) and ~19,000 patients from the Swedish Heart Failure Registry with similar performance. One of the risk factors included in all of the final models was lack of treatment with ARNI; this risk model may therefore be more appropriate for patients on contemporary GDMT, although, given its novelty, further validation in prospective cohorts will be necessary to support its clinical use.

Hospitalized Heart Failure

Although there has been progress in improving symptoms and in-hospital mortality for patients hospitalized with HF, events after discharge remain unacceptably high, with up to 15% of patients dying after discharge and 1 in 4 patients being readmitted within 90 days.[29,30] Therefore, patients with hospitalized HF (HHF) represent a high-risk group for which processes of care designed to improve outcomes with increased resources, intensive monitoring, or targeted interventions may be especially effective. However, even among patients with HHF, risk is highly variable. Several multivariable risk scores have thus been developed specifically to predict subsequent outcomes in patients hospitalized with acute decompensated HF.[31–36] Most of these scores focus on short-term outcomes of in-hospital mortality or short-term mortality or readmission after discharge. Unlike risk models for chronic ambulatory HF, predictors of outcomes for patients with HHF are more varied, although a few risk factors (namely age, SBP, and renal indices) are shared by many of these models.

In-hospital mortality

A few popular clinical risk scores have focused on the outcome of in-hospital mortality, including the Acute Decompensated Heart Failure National Registry (ADHERE) classification and regression tree (CART) model,[4] Organized Program to Initiate Lifesaving Treatment in Hospitalized Patients With Heart Failure (OPTIMIZE-HF) nomogram,[37] and Get With the Guidelines–Heart Failure (GWTG-HF) score.[5] The ADHERE CART model was derived in a large national registry of ~33,000 patient records with HHF and validated in another ~33,000 patient records using a temporal validation scheme. The resulting ADHERE CART model is a simple tool for risk assessment at the bedside using only 3 predictive variables: blood urea nitrogen (BUN), SBP, and serum creatinine. The discriminatory power of this score was modest (AUC 0.67–0.69 in derivation and validation cohorts); however, its allure lies in its simplicity and ease of use at the bedside. The OPTIMIZE-HF nomogram was derived from another national hospital-based registry of almost 50,000 patients in more than 250 hospitals. A simplified nomogram for predicting in-hospital mortality was developed using the top 8 predictors from a multivariable LR model and a separate nomogram was later developed for postdischarge outcomes of 60-day mortality and 60-day mortality or HF hospitalization.[38] The in-hospital mortality nomogram showed good discrimination with internal validation by bootstrapped resampling (AUC 0.753) as well as in external validation cohorts from the OPTIME-CHF clinical trial (AUC 0.756) and the ADHERE clinical registry (AUC 0.746). However, performance was worse for postdischarge nomograms, particularly for the prediction of HF readmission within 60 days. The GWTG-HF Score was derived from a more contemporary registry of approximately 40,000 patients with both HFrEF and HFpEF using a multivariable LR model and internally validated in a subset of the patients from this same registry. Like the ADHERE CART model, age, SBP, and BUN were the strongest contributors to risk of in-hospital mortality, whereas heart rate, presence of chronic obstructive pulmonary disease, and serum Na were weaker predictors in the final model. The model had good discriminatory power in both derivation and validation cohorts (AUC ~ 0.75) regardless of baseline left ventricle systolic function. Calibration plots revealed that the model overestimated risk of mortality in high-risk patients.

Postdischarge outcomes

Although assessing risk of adverse inpatient outcomes may help triage patients who require more immediate attention or intensive monitoring/treatment while hospitalized, postdischarge outcomes remain the greatest source of morbidity in patients with HHF. Thus, predicting postdischarge outcomes may be more consequential.

Clinical risk prediction models for postdischarge outcomes in patients with HHF have focused on outcomes of all-cause mortality, cardiovascular mortality, all-cause readmission, readmission for HF or cardiovascular causes, or composite end points of these outcomes.

The Enhanced Feedback for Effective Cardiac Treatment (EFFECT) and The Evaluation Study of Congestive Heart Failure and Pulmonary Artery Catheterization Effectiveness (ESCAPE) risk scores focused on the outcome of postdischarge mortality. The EFFECT model was derived from a retrospective community-based cohort of 4031 patients at multiple hospitals in Canada using a multivariable LR model. Predictors of mortality at both 30 days and 1 year were similar, and a composite risk score was able to adequately discriminate very-low-risk (8% mortality at 1 year) from high-risk (79% mortality at 1 year) patients with adequate discrimination in the derivation (AUC = 0.77) and internal validation (AUC = 0.76) cohorts. The ESCAPE risk score was derived from a North American clinical trial cohort of 433 patients using a Cox proportional hazards model. A simplified risk score for mortality at 6 months was constructed using 8 clinical variables with integer values assigned for each variable's contribution to the overall risk, with BUN and brain natriuretic peptide (BNP) being the most important variables in the model. The model showed good discrimination in derivation (AUC = 0.76) and internal validation with bootstrapping (AUC = 0.78) cohorts, but, when externally validated in a clinical trial cohort from the FIRST (Flolan International Randomized Survival Trial) study (without values for BNP or diuretic use available), performed much worse (AUC = 0.65).

In general, models designed to predict nonfatal end points such as readmissions perform worse than those models designed to predict mortality. In addition, predictors of mortality are typically different than those for readmissions, which may reflect the complexity of clinical and nonclinical factors that contribute to risk of hospital readmission and suggests that there may be risk factors that have not yet been identified or that are simply not captured in contemporary datasets. For example, the OPTIME-CHF (Outcomes of a Prospective Trial of Intravenous Milrinone for Exacerbations of Chronic Heart Failure) clinical trial cohort of 949 patients was used to derive 2 separate models to predict 60-day mortality or the composite of death and rehospitalization at 60 days.[9] The model for predicting mortality had better discriminatory power (AUC 0.77) than the model for predicting the composite end point

(AUC 0.69). Similarly, the Placebo-Controlled Randomized Study of the Selective A1 Adenosine Receptor Antagonist Rolofylline for Patients Hospitalized With Acute Decompensated Heart Failure and Volume Overload to Assess Treatment Effect on Congestion and Renal Function (PROTECT)–derived risk models for 30-day mortality (AUC 0.79) and 180-day mortality (AUC 0.74) performed better overall than those for predicting 30-day all-cause mortality or hospitalization (AUC 0.66) and 30-day death or hospitalization for cardiovascular reasons (AUC 0.66).[39] More recently, the BIOSTAT-CHF project was developed specifically to derive and validate risk prediction models from a large European cohort of 2516 patients across 69 hospital centers in 11 countries.[40] Although this cohort did not exclusively include patients with HHF, most patients were enrolled during an admission for worsening HF. Risk models for predicting outcomes of mortality, hospitalization for HF, and the composite outcome of these end points were derived from multivariable backward stepwise Cox proportional hazards regression models and validated in an external cohort of 1738 patients from Scotland. Discriminatory power for the mortality model (AUC 0.73) was remarkably better than for the HF hospitalization model (AUC 0.64) in the external validation cohort, and predictors included in respective models were markedly different (see **Table 2**).

Heart Failure with Preserved Ejection Fraction

All of the aforementioned risk models either excluded patients with HFpEF or were derived from mixed populations of HFrEF and HFpEF enrolled in clinical trials, registries, or community cohorts. HFpEF is an increasingly common cause of HF hospitalization in an aging population.[41] Moreover, the clinical characteristics of patients with HFpEF are distinct; risk models derived from mixed cohorts may fail to capture unique risk factors that contribute to adverse outcomes in this population.[41–44] Risk scores that have been developed specifically for patients with HFpEF are lacking, although there are a few models that warrant mention.

The I-PRESERVE score was derived from the Irbesartan in Heart Failure with Preserved Ejection Fraction clinical trial cohort of 4128 patients with chronic HFpEF using a forward selection stepwise multivariable Cox proportional hazards model for predicting the outcomes of all-cause mortality, all-cause mortality or HF hospitalization, and HF death or hospitalization.[45] Interestingly, the variables included in the final derived models are quite similar to those included in the models developed in other chronic HF cohorts discussed previously (see **Table 2**). The model was internally validated with bootstrapped resampling with good discrimination (AUC 0.711–0.765), but was not externally validated and has not been directly compared with other risk scores for chronic HF. In contrast, the Atherosclerosis Risk in Communities (ARIC) study–derived risk score was developed to specifically predict outcomes among patients with HFpEF hospitalized with acute decompensated HF.[46] The investigators used a unique approach to build their model using the previously validated EFFECT score (modified to include variables available in the ARIC cohort) as a baseline and evaluating additional candidate variables that further improved prognostication of 28-day or 1-year mortality risk. The final model included several variables that were related to comorbidities implicated in the pathophysiology of the HFpEF syndrome. This model had good discrimination in an internal validation cohort (AUC 0.73 for 28-day and 0.71 for 1-year mortality) with a modest improvement over the EFFECT model alone (AUC 0.70 for 28-day and 0.68 for 1-year mortality). Given the evolving landscape of HF and the epidemiologic impact of HFpEF, future research is clearly warranted to further refine risk prediction in this population.

LACK OF EVIDENCE FOR CLINICAL UTILITY OF RISK PREDICTION MODELS

The literature is teeming with HF risk prediction models; however, there is little evidence that incorporating risk prediction into clinical practice influences management or improves outcomes. Model development for the sake of prediction has become a popular educational hobby,[47] but, in order for risk models to be used to improve processes of care, they should be interpretable and actionable. Most models include risk factors that are not modifiable (eg, age) and it is unclear what, if any, interventions could be implemented to alter prognosis in patients identified as high risk. In addition, it is unclear what thresholds of risk should be considered high or whether there are meaningful thresholds for intervention. Specific interventions to improve adherence to therapies of proven benefit, multidisciplinary disease management programs, and transitional hospital discharge programs have shown promise in improving outcomes (particularly reduction of readmission rates) for patients hospitalized with HF in general,[48–54] but whether basing these interventions on prognostic information derived from risk models provides any incremental benefit (or reduced costs/resource use) is unknown. In those circumstances where prognosis may not be appreciably altered through intervention, there is also limited evidence that risk prediction may aid in patient-centered communication regarding risk, preparation for the possibility of death from HF, or referral for advanced HF therapies or interdisciplinary palliative care.[55]

Horne and colleagues[7] recently published the results of a clinical trial of risk score–guided multidisciplinary team–based care for approximately 6000 patients hospitalized with HF in 8 hospitals from the Intermountain health care system. Patients who were deemed high risk were identified via an automated risk score calculator embedded in the electronic health record (EHR) and were managed via a distinct care pathway that included personalized changes in their inpatient care, higher-intensity postdischarge follow-up, and a more precise discharge plan than lower-risk patients. Compared with historical controls, the risk score–guided multidisciplinary care plan resulted in 21% lower 30-day readmission and 52% lower 30-day mortality among high-risk patients. Importantly, outcomes among lower-risk patients were similar in the intervention and historical control group. In addition, although inpatient costs were higher in the intervention group, this was balanced by lower postdischarge costs and, consequently, there was no difference in overall cost between intervention and control groups. This finding suggests that the risk score–guided strategy led to improved cost-efficiency in caring for patients with HHF.

Although these results are promising, this study stands alone as the only large clinical trial of its kind. Moreover, reliability of the results may be limited by the use of historical controls rather than randomization, which may have led to confounding (although this was mitigated by the use of a staged crossover design and multivariable analysis that adjusted for potential confounders). Going forward, it is crucial that the value of risk prediction modeling for improving processes of care is rigorously evaluated in randomized clinical trials. The recent high-profile failure of the hotspotting program designed to reduce spending and improve quality of care among so-called health care superutilizers underscores the importance of confirming the utility of any presupposed pragmatic intervention in randomized clinical trials before it is adopted into routine practice.[56] The Risk Evaluation and its Impact on Clinical Decision Making and Outcomes in Heart Failure (REVeAL-HF) randomized clinical trial is currently enrolling patients within the Yale New Haven Health System to evaluate the influence of an automatically generated risk prediction score pop-up in the EHR on the management and outcomes of patients with HHF.[57] It is hoped that this randomized clinical trial of risk score–based interventions is the first of many to come.

BARRIERS TO IMPLEMENTATION OF RISK PREDICTION MODELS IN CLINICAL PRACTICE AND SYSTEMS OF CARE

Despite all of the efforts to develop a well-validated risk prediction model for patients with HF, adoption of risk modeling to assess prognosis in clinical settings is low. Less than 1% of patients enrolled in a long-term HF registry were offered information regarding prognosis calculated from a risk model by their treating clinicians.[18] One major reason for this is likely the lack of evidence for the clinical utility of implementation of HF risk scores; however, there are also several putative barriers to the use of HF risk prediction scores in practice.

First, the performance of these models, especially outside of their derivation cohorts, is disappointing. HF risk models are often derived from single-center populations or clinical trial cohorts without validation in an external cohort. Given that the risk factors for adverse outcomes can vary substantially in HF cohorts with different characteristics (eg, HFrEF vs HFpEF, clinical trial vs registry, race/ethnicity, sex, and socioeconomic diversity), the derivation cohort may be very different than the cohort to which the model is applied. Moreover, models derived from historical cohorts may fail to account for the changing landscape of HF and the effect that contemporary therapies have on outcomes; it can be difficult for risk model development to keep pace with therapeutic innovation. Outcomes modeled by different risk scores are often highly variable, including all-cause mortality, cardiovascular death, all-cause hospitalizations, HF hospitalizations, and composites of these individual end points. Each of these outcomes is associated with a different set of clinical features; even the 2 major causes of death from HF, sudden cardiac death and progressive pump failure, have distinct risk factors. In addition, nonfatal events may be more difficult to predict than mortality. Clinicians must think carefully about which outcomes are important to predict and prevent; perhaps patient-centered outcomes would be a more appropriate metric. The refractory HF risk score (see **Table 2**) introduced by Allen and colleagues[58] is unique because it focused on a primary outcome of unfavorable future HRQOL (as assessed by the Kansas City Cardiomyopathy Questionnaire [KCCQ]) or death in the 6 months following admission. Not only is this a more meaningful metric to patients than readmission rates, it may also identify patients who would benefit from end-of-life discussions or palliative care referral.

Second, HF risk scores rely on multivariable statistical modeling of population data. Selection of predictors is often based on a priori knowledge of traditional clinical risk factors for the outcome of interest and/or stepwise methods for multivariable selection based on statistical significance, both of which can be problematic and result in significant bias. Predictors included in models are often based on static measurements of clinical variables, rather than taking advantage of longitudinal dynamic changes in repeated measurements of risk factors that may be informative. Moreover, traditional statistical modeling lacks the ability to model complex, unstructured multidimensional data such as raw imaging data or free text from clinical reports. Most available models also fail to indicate how missing data are handled, with even fewer using robust methods for handling missing data such as multiple imputations. In addition, popular HF prediction models ignore the presence of competing risks, such as from noncardiac death, heart transplant, or mechanical circulatory support (an especially salient issue in the advanced HF population, where competing risks are common).[59,60] Given that statistical models predict outcomes on a population level, it is unsurprising that, in practice, these scores perform poorly on an individual level. Allen and colleagues[21] found that popular HF risk models (including SHFM and MAGGIC) performed unacceptably poorly at the individual level, with most patients who died within the next year having greater than a 75% model-predicted probability of survival.

In addition, provider inertia and skepticism present a significant barrier to adoption of risk prediction models in practice, and most providers think that risk models would not change their practice or add value to their clinical evaluations.[61,62] Up to three-quarters of clinicians surveyed rarely or never use cardiovascular risk prediction scores.[61] One of the most common reasons provided for not using risk models is the inconvenience and time required to manually calculate risk scores. Although many online calculators exist for popular HF risk scores, these still require manual input of individual risk factors, which can be prohibitively time consuming, especially in the context of increasing pressures on time constraints of the clinical encounter. An effective risk score should therefore be incorporated directly into the EHR with automatic calculation, but there are few current examples of such integration. Providers also express doubts over the utility of risk prediction models, believing these models often oversimplify the risk assessment process and that their own ability to predict risk is superior to that of any model. However, there is evidence that this belief is unfounded. Both providers and patients have proved notoriously bad at predicting prognosis, with providers tending to underestimate survival and patients tending to overestimate survival.[63–65]

PROMISE OF ARTIFICIAL INTELLIGENCE FOR RISK PREDICTION IN HEART FAILURE

Rapid advances in computational power, the digital big data revolution, and innovations in mathematical algorithms have led to a recent resurgence of enthusiasm surrounding the utility of artificial intelligence in several industries. The recent popularity of artificial intelligence has been propelled by the development of novel machine learning (ML) models, which are computer algorithms designed to learn without explicit programming, instead relying on patterns and inference from data (**Fig. 1**). ML has been applied to problems throughout various fields of medicine, particularly radiology, dermatology, and pathology. The emergence of ML technologies in cardiovascular medicine is also starting.

Given the disappointing performance and barriers to use of existing risk scores for HF, there has been substantial interest in novel methods for risk stratification. ML is able to model complex multidimensional interactions within data, and ML models are designed to optimize prediction on an individual level rather than a population level.[66] Moreover, the learning aspect of ML means that these models are modular and adaptable: ML models can be updated to predict outcomes in different populations and more contemporary cohorts as newer data become available. Given that ML models are, by definition, computer programs, they are easily integrated into existing EHR and administrative systems, enabling automated calculation of risk scores toward relieving rather than increasing the burden of resource and time constraints on clinicians and health systems.

Machine Learning for Risk Prediction in Heart Failure

Although ML for risk prediction in HF populations is still in its nascence, there are several promising examples of ML-derived risk prediction algorithms that have already been developed (**Table 3**). Compared with statistically derived risk models, most ML HF risk models incorporate large amounts of features and are derived from very large datasets. Features incorporated into these models include demographic, clinical, physical

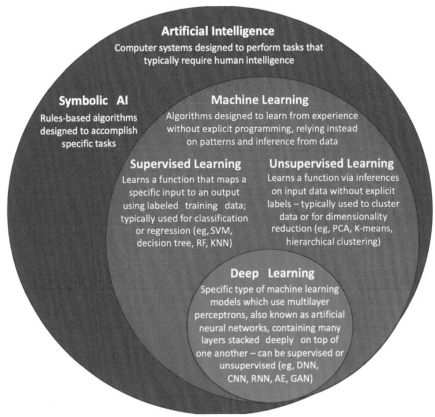

Fig. 1. Artificial intelligence and ML. Schema of the relationship between artificial intelligence, ML, and deep learning. AI, artificial intelligence; CNN, convolutional neural network; DNN, deep neural network; GAN, generative adversarial network; KNN, k-nearest neighbor; PCA, principal components analysis; RF, random forests; RNN, recurrent neural network; SVM, support vector machines.

examination, laboratory, electrocardiogram (ECG), echocardiographic, medication, procedure, hemodynamic, socioeconomic, quality-of-life, and administrative claims-based data. In addition, most of these ML-based HF risk models used cross-validation only to assess model performance, with very few using a hold-out validation set and none evaluating model performance in a completely independent test set after training was complete.

Most efforts to develop an ML-derived HF risk model have used supervised learning algorithms. Several investigators have compared HF risk prediction models derived using supervised learning with traditional statistical methodology (namely LR). Some investigators have found that ML models provided no improvement compared with LR, whereas others found modest improvement for ML compared with LR. Typically, the highest-performing ML models are derived from algorithms using ensembles of decision trees, including random forests (RFs) and gradient boosting machines (GBMs). However, even the best-

performing ML models showed discriminative power (AUC 0.62–0.73) and calibration for prediction of mortality and readmission that is on par with previously reported statistical models in the literature.

Shah and colleagues[67] used a combined approach of unsupervised and supervised learning to identify distinct phenotypes, then predict risk of disease outcomes among a cohort of 397 patients with HFpEF. Clinical, laboratory, ECG, and echocardiographic data were prospectively collected from 397 patients with HFpEF enrolled in an observational study at a single institution. A total of 46 continuous features (after filtering those that were highly correlated) were used in a penalized model-based clustering algorithm. From this analysis, 3 clinically distinct phenotypes of HFpEF were identified, each with significantly different risks of mortality or cardiovascular hospitalization. In addition, using the supervised learning technique of support vector machines, a model that included the initial 46 features plus the derived phenogroup feature had fair discriminative ability in predicting the composite outcome of HF

Table 3
Machine learning models for predicting outcomes in patients with heart failure

Study	Population	Target (Outcomes)	Features (Predictors)	Models	Performance	Validation/Test Sets
Shah et al,[67] 2015	Recently hospitalized outpatients with HFpEF: N = 420	CV hosp, HF hosp, and death	46 features: clinical variables, physical characteristics, laboratory tests, ECG, and echocardiogram parameters	Phenomapping via model-based clustering + risk prediction via SVM	Combined model AUC 0.67 for primary outcome	Hold-out validation: 107 patients with HFpEF
Loghma-npour et al,[138] 2016	Pre-LVAD patients: N = 10,909	Right ventricular failure after LVAD	33 features: preoperative demographics, clinical features, laboratory tests, echocardiogram, hemodynamics, others	Tree-augmented naive bayesian network	AUC 0.903 for acute RVF (vs Drakos 0.547 and RVFRS 0.498)	10-fold cross-validation
Mortazavi et al,[139] 2016	Recently discharged patients with HF: N = 1653	30-d and 180-d all-cause readmission and readmission for HF	236 features: demographics, laboratory tests, physical examination, quality of life, SES	RF, GBM, RF/SVM, RF/LR vs LR	All-cause hosp: RF (best) (AUC 0.628 vs 0.533 LR) HF hosp: GBM (best) (AUC 0.678 vs 0.543 LR)	50% random hold-out validation
Frizzel et al,[140] 2017	Inpatients with HF from GWTG-HF registry: N = 56,477	30-d all-cause readmission	86 features: demographics, SES, medical history, characterization of HF, medications, vital signs, weights, laboratory tests, treatment, and discharge interventions	Tree-augmented naive bayesian network, LR with LASSO, RF, and GBM	AUC 0.607–0.618 vs 0.624 for LR	30% random hold-out validation
Ahmad et al,[141] 2018	Swedish HF	1-y survival	86 features: demographics,	RF, K-means clustering (using top 8 features from RF)	RF AUC 0.83, 8 cluster variables AUC 0.78	10-fold cross-validation

Source	Population	Outcome	Features	Model	Results	Validation
	registry—N = 44,886 clinical, laboratory, and imaging data					
Golas et al,[142] 2018	Patients with a history of HF admission: N = 11,510	30-d all-cause readmission	3512 features: demographics, admissions, diagnosis, procedure, medication, and laboratory data; unstructured text data from clinical notes	Deep unified neural networks, bag-of-words model for text	AUC 0.705 vs 0.664 for LR	10-fold cross-validation
Adler et al,[143] 2019	Patients with initial occurrence of HF: N = 5882	Death within 90 d (high-risk) or no HF event after 800 d (low risk)	8 features: DBP, Cr, BUN, Hgb, WBC, platelets, albumin, RDW	GBM	AUC 0.88 (0.81 and 0.84 in external test cohorts)	50% random hold-out validation, external test sets in 2 separate cohorts
Angraal et al,[144] 2019	Outpatients with HFpEF in TOPCAT: N = 1767	All-cause mortality and HF hosp through 3-y follow-up	86 features: demographic, clinical, laboratory, and electrocardiography data; KCCQ scores	LR with LASSO, RF, GBM, SVM	RF (best): AUC 0.72 mortality and 0.76 HF hosp (vs 0.66 and 0.73 for LRR)	5-fold cross-validation
Desai et al,[145] 2020	Patients with HF by Medicare claims: N = 9502	Mortality, HF hosp, high cost, home days lost	54 features: demographics, HF-related variables, medications, comorbidities, and claims-based frailty index and SES index	LR with LASSO, CART, RF, GBM	AUC for GBM (best) vs LR Mortality 0.727 vs 0.7124 HF hosp 0.745 vs 0.707 High cost 0.733 vs 0.734 Home days lost 0.790 vs 0.781	10-fold cross-validation, hold-out test set 3389 patients

Abbreviations: ECG, electrocardiogram; GBM, gradient boosting machine; LASSO, least absolute shrinkage and selection operator; RDW, red cell distribution width; RF, random forest; SES, socioeconomic status; SVM, support vector machine.

hospitalization, cardiovascular hospitalization, or death (AUC 0.67). Ahmad and colleagues[68] also used a combined approach to develop a risk prediction model among patients in the Swedish Heart Failure Registry by applying supervised learning before unsupervised learning to model risk. First, an RFs algorithm was used to identify predictors of 1-year survival. Discrimination based on the full RFs model (AUC 0.828) was excellent and higher than that historically reported in popular statistical models for predicting 1-year mortality (eg, SHFM and MAGGIC). Next, unsupervised learning via K-means clustering was applied to the 8 most predictive features identified from the supervised learning algorithm to identify 4 clinically relevant subgroups of HF with distinct risk profiles. Patients in the highest-risk cluster had only a 69% 1-year survival, compared with 93% 1-year survival in the lowest-risk group. There are a few other recent examples in the literature of unsupervised learning to identify clusters of patients with distinct risk profiles for clinically meaningful outcomes among patients with chronic HF and those hospitalized with acute decompensated HF.

Limitations of Machine Learning Risk Models

Thus far, the authors have yet to see any real adoption of ML risk models for HF in clinical practice or systems of care. ML-derived risk models have generally failed to live up to inflated expectations, showing only modest improvement compared with traditional statistical models. Although some of these shortcomings may simply be caused by the fallacy of believing that the future can be predicted, there are other considerations regarding the potential pitfalls and limitations of ML risk models that should be noted.

Many of the problems that have plagued their statistical predecessors have also troubled ML-derived models. Existing ML models for risk prediction in HF have generally failed to account adequately for time to event outcomes, competing risks, or missing data, although strategies and algorithms to address these problems exist and research in this area is active.[69,70] In addition, most ML models use discrete values from a single time point as input features, ignoring the predictive ability of longitudinal data that change over time. Many ML models have an exceptional ability to analyze time-series data and adjust risk probabilities as new information becomes available, thereby accounting for some of the intrinsically stochastic nature of risk prediction. Further, clinicians should not expect any significant performance boost from simply using a novel methodology for analyzing data when using the same features/predictors (demographics, vital signs, laboratory tests) that were typically used in statistical models.[71] One of the strengths of the complexity of ML models, particularly deep learning models, is the ability to handle complex, raw data as inputs as long as the quantity of data is sufficient for the model to learn meaningful representations.[72]

There are also new considerations presented by ML techniques. Given their complexity, ML models are prone to overfitting to training data, which can limit the ability to generalize to external datasets.[66,72] It is therefore crucial that any ML model is validated multiple times in independent datasets before being adopted for clinical use. Moreover, there are concerns regarding the interpretability of ML models because they can be perceived as being a black box because of their focus on the result of the model rather than transparency of the model itself.[73] Further, ML models often consider thousands of features so it may be difficult to decide which risk factors are most important and, consequently, how clinicians could intervene to modify this risk. To address these concerns, new visualization techniques are being developed in order to codify the importance of individual features in ML algorithms (eg, heat-map visualization of layer class activation in convolutional neural networks) and make these models more actionable.[74] As with statistically derived risk models, randomized clinical trials assessing the influence of using ML-based HF risk modeling on management and clinically important outcomes are imperative.

In addition, the era of ML brings new cultural and sociologic concerns that should be noted.[73] ML models, particularly supervised learning models, often rely on massive amounts of well-labeled data that require a significant degree of human input, although there are many strategies to reduce this reliance on human microwork, such as semisupervised learning, data augmentation, transfer learning, fine-tuning, and feature extraction. There is also inherent risk in introducing human implicit bias when developing an ML model, and there are countless examples of unintended and often discriminatory results of ML models.[75] In addition, the human-machine interface has become an important consideration, and popular culture has promoted a general fear and resistance to the adoption of these technologies that can be perceived to be replacing human input, especially among health care providers. However, there are abundant examples in the literature that augmented intelligence (ie, a human being with the assistance of an artificially intelligent system) almost always outperforms a human or machine alone.[71]

SUMMARY AND FUTURE DIRECTIONS

Predicting outcomes in patients with HF has proved difficult. Although many individual risk factors for adverse future outcomes are known, attempts at developing high-performing risk models in various HF populations using statistically based methods have generally underwhelming. Moreover, there is currently a lack of evidence to support the notion that implementation of these risk scores into clinical practice or systems of care improves outcomes. Newer methods of risk prediction using ML technologies offer promise, but thus far have failed to live up to the hype of expectations.

Although artificial intelligence may play a role in the future of risk prediction in HF, many key challenges remain. Clinicians must think more broadly about the predictors or features included in risk models, including source data from unstructured clinical notes text, imaging, pathology slides, hemodynamic and ECG tracings, sensor data (ambulatory monitors, pulmonary artery sensors, and consumer wearables), and other omics data (genomics, proteomics, metabolomics, and so forth). More robust models can be built using agnostic deep learning algorithms, and perhaps the key to predicting the as-yet unpredictable is in some of the unrecognized or hidden features in these raw data. In addition, future research is needed to develop better strategies to communicate risk to patients and families in a way that enhances comprehension, identify clinically meaningful thresholds to implement clinical action items (eg, telemonitoring, pulmonary artery pressure monitoring, multidisciplinary care initiatives), and rigorously evaluate risk score–based strategies in randomized clinical trials. Clinicians should strive to constantly assess for bias and ensure that risk models are both equitable and actionable on an individual level; that they are not just predicting the future but are able to intervene and change that future.

DISCLOSURE

S.J. Shah is supported by grants from the National Institutes of Health (R01 HL140731, R01 HL120728, R01 HL107577, and R01 HL149423); the American Heart Association (#16SFRN28780016, #15CVGPSD27260148); Actelion, AstraZeneca, Corvia, and Novartis; and has received consulting fees from Actelion, Amgen, AstraZeneca, Bayer, Boehringer-Ingelheim, Cardiora, Eisai, Ionis, Ironwood, Merck, Novartis, Pfizer, Sanofi, and United Therapeutics. F.S. Ahmad is supported in part by a grant from the Agency for Healthcare Research and Quality (K12 HS026385) and has received consulting fees from Amgen. S.S. Khan is supported by a grant from the National Institutes of Health/National Heart, Lung, and Blood Institute (KL2TR001424). The other authors have nothing to disclose.

REFERENCES

1. Virani SS, Alonso A, Benjamin EJ, et al, WRITING GROUP MEMBERS On behalf of the American Heart Association Council on Epidemiology and Prevention Statistics Committee and Stroke Statistics Subcommittee. Heart Disease and Stroke Statistics-2020 Update A Report From the American Heart Association. Circulation 2020;141(9): e139–596.

2. Yancy CW, Jessup M, Bozkurt B, et al. 2013 ACCF/ AHA guideline for the management of heart failure: A report of the american college of cardiology foundation/american heart association task force on practice guidelines. Circulation 2013;128(16). https://doi.org/10.1161/CIR.0b013e31829e8776.

3. Heidenreich PA, Albert NM, Allen LA, et al. Forecasting the impact of heart failure in the united states a policy statement from the american heart association. Circ Heart Fail 2013;6(3):606–19.

4. Fonarow GC, Adams KF, Abraham WT, et al. Risk stratification for in-hospital mortality in acutely decompensated heart failure: Classification and regression tree analysis. J Am Med Assoc 2005; 293(5):572–80.

5. Peterson PN, Rumsfeld JS, Liang L, et al. A validated risk score for in-hospital mortality in patients with heart failure from the American heart association get with the guidelines program. Circ Cardiovasc Qual Outcomes 2010;3(1):25–32.

6. O'Connor CM, Hasselblad V, Mehta RH, et al. Triage after hospitalization with advanced heart failure. The ESCAPE (evaluation study of congestive heart failure and pulmonary artery catheterization effectiveness) risk model and discharge score. J Am Coll Cardiol 2010;55(9):872–8.

7. Horne BD, Roberts CA, Rasmusson KD, et al. Risk score–guided multidisciplinary team-based Care for Heart Failure Inpatients is associated with lower 30-day readmission and lower 30-day mortality. Am Heart J 2020;219:78–88.

8. Prasad H, Sra J, Levy WC, et al. Influence of predictive modeling in implementing optimal heart failure therapy. Am J Med Sci 2011;341(3):185–90.

9. Felker GM, Leimberger JD, Califf RM, et al. Risk stratification after hospitalization for decompensated heart failure. J Card Fail 2004;10(6): 460–6.

10. Collins GS, Reitsma JB, Altman DG, et al. Transparent Reporting of a multivariable prediction model for Individual Prognosis Or Diagnosis (TRIPOD): The TRIPOD Statement. Ann Intern Med 2015;162(1):55.

11. Moons KGM, Altman DG, Reitsma JB, et al. Transparent reporting of a multivariable prediction model for individual prognosis or diagnosis (TRIPOD): Explanation and elaboration. Ann Intern Med 2015;162(1):W1–73.

12. Lloyd-Jones DM. Cardiovascular risk prediction: Basic concepts, current status, and future directions. Circulation 2010;121(15):1768–77.

13. Hickey GL, Blackstone EH. External model validation of binary clinical risk prediction models in cardiovascular and thoracic surgery. J Thorac Cardiovasc Surg 2016;152(2):351–5.

14. Rahimi K, Bennett D, Conrad N, et al. Risk prediction in patients with heart failure: A systematic review and analysis. JACC Hear Fail 2014;2(5):440–6.

15. Di Tanna GL, Wirtz H, Burrows KL, et al. Evaluating risk prediction models for adults with heart failure: A systematic literature review. PLoS One 2020; 15(1):e0224135.

16. Ouwerkerk W, Voors AA, Zwinderman AH. Factors influencing the predictive power of models for predicting mortality and/or heart failure hospitalization inpatients with heart failure. JACC Hear Fail 2014; 2(5):429–36.

17. Alba AC, Agoritsas T, Jankowski M, et al. Risk prediction models for mortality in ambulatory patients with heart failure a systematic review. Circ Heart Fail 2013;6(5):881–9.

18. Canepa M, Fonseca C, Chioncel O, et al. Performance of prognostic risk scores in chronic heart failure patients enrolled in the european society of cardiology heart failure long-term registry. JACC Hear Fail 2018;6(6):452–62.

19. Levy WC, Mozaffarian D, Linker DT, et al. The Seattle heart failure model: prediction of survival in heart failure. Circulation 2006;113(11):1424–33.

20. Packer M, O'Connor CM, Ghali JK, et al. Effect of amlodipine on morbidity and mortality in severe chronic heart failure. N Engl J Med 1996;335(15): 1107–14.

21. Allen LA, Matlock DD, Shetterly SM, et al. Use of risk models to predict death in the next year among individual ambulatory patients with heart failure. JAMA Cardiol 2017;2(4):435–41.

22. Pocock SJ, Ariti CA, McMurray JJV, et al. Predicting survival in heart failure: A risk score based on 39 372 patients from 30 studies. Eur Heart J 2013;34(19):1404–13.

23. Sartipy U, Dahlström U, Edner M, et al. Predicting survival in heart failure: Validation of the MAGGIC heart failure risk score in 51 043 patients from the Swedish Heart Failure Registry. Eur J Heart Fail 2014;16(2):173–9.

24. Rich JD, Burns J, Freed BH, et al. Meta-analysis global group in chronic (MAGGIC) heart failure risk score: Validation of a simple tool for the prediction of morbidity and mortality in heart failure with preserved ejection fraction. J Am Heart Assoc 2018;7(20):1–12.

25. Pocock SJ, Wang D, Pfeffer MA, et al. Predictors of mortality and morbidity in patients with chronic heart failure. Eur Heart J 2006;27(1):65–75.

26. Wedel H, McMurray JJV, Lindberg M, et al. Predictors of fatal and non-fatal outcomes in the Controlled Rosuvastatin Multinational Trial in Heart Failure (CORONA): Incremental value of apolipoprotein A-1, high-sensitivity C-reactive peptide and N-terminal pro B-type natriuretic peptide. Eur J Heart Fail 2009;11(3):281–91.

27. Barlera S, Tavazzi L, Franzosi MG, et al. Predictors of mortality in 6975 patients with chronic heart failure in the gruppo italiano per lo studio della streptochinasi nell'infarto miocardico-heart failure trial proposal for a nomogram. Circ Heart Fail 2013;6(1):31–9.

28. Simpson J, Jhund PS, Lund LH, et al. Prognostic Models Derived in PARADIGM-HF and Validated in ATMOSPHERE and the Swedish Heart Failure Registry to predict mortality and morbidity in chronic heart failure. JAMA Cardiol 2020;1–10. https://doi.org/10.1001/jamacardio.2019.5850.

29. Bueno H, Ross JS, Wang Y, et al. Trends in length of stay and short-term outcomes among medicare patients hospitalized for heart failure, 1993-2006. JAMA 2010;303(21):2141–7.

30. Gheorghiade M, Shah AN, Vaduganathan M, et al. Recognizing hospitalized heart failure as an entity and developing new therapies to improve outcomes. academics', clinicians', industry's, regulators', and payers' perspectives. Heart Fail Clin 2013;9(3):285–90.

31. Ross JS, Mulvey GK, Stauffer B, et al. Statistical models and patient predictors of readmission for heart failure: A systematic review. Arch Intern Med 2008;168(13):1371–86.

32. Fonarow GC. Clinical risk prediction tools in patients hospitalized with heart failure. Rev Cardiovasc Med 2012;13(1):14–23.

33. Passantino A. Predicting mortality in patients with acute heart failure: Role of risk scores. World J Cardiol 2015;7(12):902.

34. Saito M, Negishi K, Marwick TH. Meta-analysis of risks for short-term readmission in patients with heart failure. Am J Cardiol 2016;117(4):626–32.

35. Lagu T, Pekow PS, Shieh MS, et al. Validation and comparison of seven mortality prediction models for hospitalized patients with acute decompensated heart failure. Circ Heart Fail 2016;9(8):1–10.

36. Mahajan SM, Heidenreich P, Abbott B, et al. Predictive models for identifying risk of readmission after index hospitalization for heart failure: A systematic review. Eur J Cardiovasc Nurs 2018. https://doi.org/10.1177/1474515118799059.

37. Abraham WT, Fonarow GC, Albert NM, et al. Predictors of in-hospital mortality in patients

hospitalized for heart failure. insights from the organized program to initiate lifesaving treatment in hospitalized patients with heart failure (OPTIMIZE-HF). J Am Coll Cardiol 2008;52(5):347–56.

38. O'Connor CM, Abraham WT, Albert NM, et al. Predictors of mortality after discharge in patients hospitalized with heart failure: An analysis from the Organized Program to Initiate Lifesaving Treatment in Hospitalized Patients with Heart Failure (OPTIMIZE-HF). Am Heart J 2008;156(4):662–73.

39. Cleland JG, Chiswell K, Teerlink JR, et al. Predictors of postdischarge outcomes from information acquired shortly after admission for acute heart failure: A report from the placebo-controlled randomized study of the selective a1 adenosine receptor antagonist rolofylline for patients hospitalized w. Circ Heart Fail 2014;7(1):76–87.

40. Voors AA, Ouwerkerk W, Zannad F, et al. Development and validation of multivariable models to predict mortality and hospitalization in patients with heart failure. Eur J Heart Fail 2017;19(5):627–34.

41. Steinberg BA, Zhao X, Heidenreich PA, et al. Trends in patients hospitalized with heart failure and preserved left ventricular ejection fraction: Prevalence, therapies, and outcomes. Circulation 2012;126(1):65–75.

42. Vaduganathan M, Fonarow GC. Epidemiology of hospitalized heart failure. differences and similarities between patients with reduced versus preserved ejection fraction. Heart Fail Clin 2013;9(3):271–6.

43. Doughty RN, Cubbon R, Ezekowitz J, et al. The survival of patients with heart failure with preserved or reduced left ventricular ejection fraction: An individual patient data meta-analysis: Meta-analysis Global Group in Chronic Heart Failure (MAGGIC). Eur Heart J 2013;33(14):1750–7.

44. Kapoor JR, Kapoor R, Ju C, et al. Precipitating clinical factors, heart failure characterization, and outcomes in patients hospitalized with heart failure with reduced, borderline, and preserved ejection fraction. JACC Hear Fail 2016;4(6):464–72.

45. Komajda M, Carson PE, Hetzel S, et al. Factors associated with outcome in heart failure with preserved ejection fraction. Circ Heart Fail 2011;4(1):27–35.

46. Thorvaldsen T, Claggett BL, Shah A, et al. Predicting risk in patients hospitalized for acute decompensated heart failure and preserved ejection fraction: the atherosclerosis risk in communities study heart failure community surveillance. Circ Heart Fail 2017;10(12):1–10.

47. Stevenson LW, Davis RB. Model building as an educational hobby. Circ Heart Fail 2016;9(8). https://doi.org/10.1161/CIRCHEARTFAILURE.116.003457.

48. Ahmad FS, Metlay JP, Barg FK, et al. Identifying hospital organizational strategies to reduce readmissions. Am J Med Qual 2013;28(4):278–85.

49. McAlister FA, Stewart S, Ferrua S, et al. Multidisciplinary strategies for the management of heart failure patients at high risk for admission: A systematic review of randomized trials. J Am Coll Cardiol 2004;44(4):810–9.

50. Holland R, Battersby J, Harvey I, et al. Systematic review of multidisciplinary interventions in heart failure. Heart 2005;91(7):899–906.

51. Murray MD, Young J, Hoke S, et al. Pharmacist intervention to improve medication adherence in heart failure: A randomized trial. Ann Intern Med 2007;146(10):714–25.

52. Granger BB, Ekman I, Hernandez AF, et al. Results of the chronic heart failure intervention to improve medication adherence study: A randomized intervention in high-risk patients. Am Heart J 2015;169(4):539–48.

53. McAlister FA, Lawson FME, Teo KK, et al. A systematic review of randomized trials of disease management programs in heart failure. Am J Med 2001;110(5):378–84.

54. Peiris D, Usherwood T, Panaretto K, et al. Effect of a computer-guided, quality improvement program for cardiovascular disease risk management in primary health care: The treatment of cardiovascular risk using electronic decision support cluster-randomized trial. Circ Cardiovasc Qual Outcomes 2015;8(1):87–95.

55. Rogers JG, Patel CB, Mentz RJ, et al. Palliative care in heart failure: the PAL-HF randomized, controlled clinical trial. J Am Coll Cardiol 2017. https://doi.org/10.1016/j.jacc.2017.05.030.

56. Finkelstein A, Zhou A, Taubman S, et al. Health care hotspotting - A randomized, controlled trial. N Engl J Med 2020;382(2):152–62.

57. Tariq Ahmad MM, Nihar R, Desai MM, et al. Risk EValuation And Its Impact on ClinicAL Decision Making and Outcomes in Heart Failure (REVeAL-HF). ClinicalTrials.gov. Available at: https://clinicaltrials.gov/ct2/show/NCT03845660. Accessed February 5, 2020.

58. Allen LA, Gheorghiade M, Reid KJ, et al. Identifying patients hospitalized with heart failure at risk for unfavorable future quality of life. Circ Cardiovasc Qual Outcomes 2011;4(4):389–98.

59. Fang J, Abdel-Qadir H, Austin PC, et al. Importance of considering competing risks in time-to-event analyses. Circ Cardiovasc Qual Outcomes 2018;11(7). https://doi.org/10.1161/circoutcomes.118.004580.

60. Austin PC, Lee DS, Fine JP. Introduction to the analysis of survival data in the presence of competing risks. Circulation 2016;133(6):601–9.

61. Eichler K, Zoller M, Tschudi P, et al. Barriers to apply cardiovascular prediction rules in primary care: A postal survey. BMC Fam Pract 2007;8. https://doi.org/10.1186/1471-2296-8-1.

62. Sposito AC, Ramires JAF, Wouter Jukema J, et al. Physicians' attitudes and adherence to use of risk scores for primary prevention of cardiovascular disease: Cross-sectional survey in three world regions. Curr Med Res Opin 2009;25(5):1171–8.

63. Yamokoski LM, Hasselblad V, Moser DK, et al. Prediction of rehospitalization and death in severe heart failure by physicians and nurses of the ESCAPE trial. J Card Fail 2007;13(1):8–13.

64. Allen LA, Yager JE, Funk MJ, et al. Discordance between patient-predicted and model-predicted life expectancy among ambulatory patients with heart failure. JAMA 2008;299(21):2533–42.

65. Buchan TA, Ross HJ, McDonald M, et al. Physician judgment versus model predicted prognosis in patients with heart failure. Can J Cardiol 2019;36(1):84–91.

66. Obermeyer Z, Emanuel EJ. Predicting the future-big data, machine learning, and clinical medicine. N Engl J Med 2016;375(13):1216–9.

67. Shah SJ, Katz DH, Selvaraj S, et al. Phenomapping for novel classification of heart failure with preserved ejection fraction. Circulation 2015;131(3):269–79.

68. Ahmad T, Pencina MJ, Schulte PJ, et al. Clinical implications of chronic heart failure phenotypes defined by cluster analysis. J Am Coll Cardiol 2014;64(17):1765–74.

69. Krittanawong C, Johnson KW, Rosenson RS, et al. Deep learning for cardiovascular medicine: A practical primer. Eur Heart J 2019;40(25):2058–2069C.

70. Wang P, Li Y, Reddy CK. Machine learning for survival analysis: A survey. ACM Comput Surv 2019;51(6). https://doi.org/10.1145/3214306.

71. Chen JH, Asch SM. Machine learning and prediction in medicine-beyond the peak of inflated expectations. N Engl J Med 2017;376(26):2507–9.

72. Deo RC. Machine learning in medicine. Circulation 2015;132(20):1920–30.

73. Verghese A, Shah NH, Harrington RA. What this computer needs is a physician humanism and artificial intelligence. JAMA 2018;319(1):19–20.

74. Samek W, Binder A, Montavon G, et al. Evaluating the visualization of what a deep neural network has learned. IEEE Trans Neural Netw Learn Syst 2017;28(11):2660–73.

75. Topol EJ. High-performance medicine: the convergence of human and artificial intelligence. Nat. Med 2019;25:44–56.

76. Ho KKL, Anderson KM, Kannel WB, et al. Survival after the onset of congestive heart failure in Framingham Heart Study subjects. Circulation 1993;88(1):107–15.

77. Wong CM, Hawkins NM, Jhund PS, et al. Clinical characteristics and outcomes of young and very young adults with heart failure: The CHARM programme (candesartan in heart failure assessment of reduction in mortality and morbidity). J Am Coll Cardiol 2013;62(20):1845–54.

78. Romiti GF, Recchia F, Zito A, et al. Sex and gender-related issues in heart failure. Heart Fail Clin 2020;16(1):121–30.

79. Glynn P, Lloyd-Jones DM, Feinstein MJ, et al. Disparities in cardiovascular mortality related to heart failure in the United States. J Am Coll Cardiol 2019;73(18):2354–5.

80. Akintoye E, Briasoulis A, Egbe A, et al. National trends in admission and in-hospital mortality of patients with heart failure in the United States (2001-2014). J Am Heart Assoc 2017;6(12). https://doi.org/10.1161/JAHA.117.006955.

81. Massimo P, Egidio T, Giovanni C, et al. Loading manipulations improve the prognostic value of doppler evaluation of mitral flow in patients with chronic heart failure. Circulation 1997;95(5):1222–30.

82. Felker GM, Thompson RE, Hare JM, et al. Underlying causes and long-term survival in patients with initially unexplained cardiomyopathy. N Engl J Med 2000;342(15):1077–84.

83. Taylor MRG, Fain PR, Sinagra G, et al. Natural history of dilated cardiomyopathy due to lamin A/C gene mutations. J Am Coll Cardiol 2003;41(5):771–80.

84. The Criteria Committee of the New York Heart Association. Classification of functional capacity and objective assessment. In: Dolgin Martin, editor. Nomenclature and criteria for diagnosis of diseases of the heart and great vessels. 9th edition. Boston: Little, Brown & Co; 1994. p. 253–6.

85. Goldman L, Hashimoto B, Cook EF, et al. Comparative reproducibility and validity of systems for assessing cardiovascular functional class: Advantages of a new specific activity scale. Circulation 1981;64(6):1227–34.

86. Taichman DB, McGoon MD, Harhay MO, et al. Wide variation in clinicians' assessment of New York Heart Association/World Health Organization functional class in patients with pulmonary arterial hypertension. Mayo Clin Proc 2009;84(7):586–92.

87. Hunt SA, Abraham WT, Chin MH, et al. 2009 focused update incorporated Into the ACC/AHA 2005 guidelines for the diagnosis and management of heart failure in adults. A Report of the American College of Cardiology Foundation/American Heart Association Task Force on practice guidelines developed. J Am Coll Cardiol 2009;53(15). https://doi.org/10.1016/j.jacc.2008.11.013.

88. Stevenson LW, Pagani FD, Young JB, et al. INTERMACS profiles of advanced heart failure: the current picture. J Heart Lung Transplant 2009;28(6):535–41.

89. Valentova M, Anker SD, von Haehling S. Cardiac cachexia revisited: the role of wasting in heart failure. Heart Fail Clin 2020;16(1):61–9.

90. Shindler DM, Kostis JB, Yusuf S, et al. Diabetes mellitus, a predictor of morbidity and mortality in the Studies of Left Ventricular Dysfunction (SOLVD) trials and registry. Am J Cardiol 1996;77(11):1017–20.

91. Schmidt M, Ulrichsen SP, Pedersen L, et al. Thirty-year trends in heart failure hospitalization and mortality rates and the prognostic impact of co-morbidity: A Danish nationwide cohort study. Eur J Heart Fail 2016;18(5):490–9.

92. Lawson CA, Mamas MA, Jones PW, et al. Association of medication intensity and stages of airflow limitation with the risk of hospitalization or death in patients with heart failure and chronic obstructive pulmonary disease. JAMA Netw Open 2018;1(8):e185489.

93. Xanthopoulos A, Starling RC, Kitai T, et al. Heart failure and liver disease: cardiohepatic interactions. JACC Hear Fail 2019;7(2):87–97.

94. Costanzo MR. The cardiorenal syndrome in heart failure. Heart Fail Clin 2020;16(1):81–97.

95. Lam CSP, Teng THK. Minding the gap in heart failure. Understanding the pulse pressure in reduced versus preserved ejection fraction. JACC Hear Fail 2016;4(1):50–4.

96. Chin MH, Goldman L. Correlates of early hospital readmission or death in patients with congestive heart failure. Am J Cardiol 1997;79(12):1640–4.

97. Chahal H, Bluemke DA, Wu CO, et al. Heart failure risk prediction in the multi-ethnic study of atherosclerosis. Heart 2015;101(1):58–64.

98. Lee TT, Chen J, Cohen DJ, et al. The association between blood pressure and mortality in patients with heart failure. Am Heart J 2006;151(1):76–83.

99. Fox K, Ford I, Steg PG, et al. Heart rate as a prognostic risk factor in patients with coronary artery disease and left-ventricular systolic dysfunction (BEAUTIFUL): a subgroup analysis of a randomised controlled trial. Lancet 2008;372(9641):817–21.

100. Obeidat M, Burgess M, Lip GYH. Atrial fibrillation in heart failure: focus on antithrombotic management. Heart Fail Clin 2020;16(1):107–20.

101. Linssen GCM, Rienstra M, Jaarsma T, et al. Clinical and prognostic effects of atrial fibrillation in heart failure patients with reduced and preserved left ventricular ejection fraction. Eur J Heart Fail 2011;13(10):1111–20.

102. Santhanakrishnan R, Wang N, Larson MG, et al. Atrial fibrillation begets heart failure and vice versa: Temporal associations and differences in preserved versus reduced ejection fraction. Circulation 2016;133(5):484–92.

103. Wang NC, Maggioni AP, Konstam MA, et al. Clinical implications of QRS duration in patients hospitalized with worsening heart failure and reduced left ventricular ejection fraction. JAMA 2008;299(22):2656–66.

104. Ellis ER, Josephson ME. Ventricular Arrhythmias and Heart Failure. In: Eisen H, editor. Heart failure: a comprehensive guide to pathophysiology and clinical care. London: Springer London; 2017. p. 339–69.

105. Lee WH, Packer M. Prognostic importance of serum sodium concentration and its modification by converting-enzyme inhibition in patients with severe chronic heart failure. Circulation 1986;73(2):257–67.

106. Fonarow GC, Peacock WF, Phillips CO, et al. Admission B-type natriuretic peptide levels and in-hospital mortality in acute decompensated heart failure. J Am Coll Cardiol 2007;49(19):1943–50.

107. Kociol RD, Horton JR, Fonarow GC, et al. Admission, discharge, or change in B-type natriuretic peptide and long-term outcomes: Data from Organized Program to Initiate Lifesaving Treatment in Hospitalized Patients with Heart Failure (OPTIMIZE-HF) linked to Medicare claims. Circ Heart Fail 2011;4(5):628–36.

108. Savarese G, Musella F, D'Amore C, et al. Changes of natriuretic peptides predict hospital admissions in patients with chronic heart failure. A meta-analysis. JACC Hear Fail 2014;2(2):148–58.

109. Khanam SS, Son JW, Lee JW, et al. Prognostic value of short-term follow-up BNP in hospitalized patients with heart failure. BMC Cardiovasc Disord 2017;17(1):1–10.

110. Richter B, Koller L, Hohensinner PJ, et al. A multibiomarker risk score improves prediction of long-term mortality in patients with advanced heart failure. Int J Cardiol 2013;168(2):1251–7.

111. Carluccio E, Dini FL, Biagioli P, et al. The "Echo Heart Failure Score": An echocardiographic risk prediction score of mortality in systolic heart failure. Eur J Heart Fail 2013;15(8):868–76.

112. Hamada-Harimura Y, Seo Y, Ishizu T, et al. Incremental prognostic value of right ventricular strain in patients with acute decompensated heart failure. Circ Cardiovasc Imaging 2018;11(10):e007249.

113. Park JJ, Park JB, Park JH, et al. Global longitudinal strain to predict mortality in patients with acute heart failure. J Am Coll Cardiol 2018;71(18):1947–57.

114. Marwick TH, Shah SJ, Thomas JD. Myocardial strain in the assessment of patients with heart failure: a review. JAMA Cardiol 2019;4(3):287–94.

115. Kuruvilla S, Adenaw N, Katwal AB, et al. Late gadolinium enhancement on cardiac magnetic resonance predicts adverse cardiovascular outcomes in nonischemic cardiomyopathy: A systematic

review and meta-analysis. Circ Cardiovasc Imaging 2014;7(2):250–7.

116. Halliday BP, Baksi AJ, Gulati A, et al. Outcome in dilated cardiomyopathy related to the extent, location, and pattern of late gadolinium enhancement. JACC Cardiovasc Imaging 2019;12(8P2):1645–55.

117. Craig M, Pereira NL. Right heart catheterization and risk stratification in advanced heart failure. Curr Heart Fail Rep 2006;3(3):143–52.

118. Cooper LB, Mentz RJ, Stevens SR, et al. Hemodynamic predictors of heart failure morbidity and mortality: fluid or flow? J Card Fail 2016;22(3):182–9.

119. Gregg F. Treatment targets in heart failure continued hemodynamics in decompensated heart failure. Rev Cardiovasc Med 2001;2(suppl 2): s7–12. Available at: http://medreviews.com/sites/default/files/2016-11/RICM_2suppl2_s7.pdf.

120. Nohria A, Tsang SW, Fang JC, et al. Clinical assessment identifies hemodynamic profiles that predict outcomes in patients admitted with heart failure. J Am Coll Cardiol 2003;41(10):1797–804.

121. Ghio S, Gavazzi A, Campana C, et al. Independent and additive prognostic value of right ventricular systolic function and pulmonary artery pressure in patients with chronic heart failure. J Am Coll Cardiol 2001;37(1):183–8.

122. Patel CB, Devore AD, Felker GM, et al. Characteristics and outcomes of patients with heart failure and discordant findings by right-sided heart catheterization and cardiopulmonary exercise testing. Am J Cardiol 2014;114(7):1059–64.

123. Borlaug BA, Nishimura RA, Sorajja P, et al. Exercise hemodynamics enhance diagnosis of early heart failure with preserved ejection fraction. Circ Heart Fail 2010;3(5):588–95.

124. Methvin A, Georgiopoulou VV, Kalogeropoulos AP, et al. Usefulness of cardiac index and peak exercise oxygen consumption for determining priority for cardiac transplantation. Am J Cardiol 2010; 105(9):1353–5.

125. Myers J, Wong M, Adhikarla C, et al. Cardiopulmonary and noninvasive hemodynamic responses to exercise predict outcomes in heart failure. J Card Fail 2013;19(2):101–7.

126. Keteyian SJ, Patel M, Kraus WE, et al. Variables measured during cardiopulmonary exercise testing as predictors of mortality in chronic systolic heart failure. J Am Coll Cardiol 2016;67(7):780–9.

127. Setoguchi S, Stevenson LW, Schneeweiss S. Repeated hospitalizations predict mortality in the community population with heart failure. Am Heart J 2007;154(2):260–6.

128. Krumholz HM, Chen YT, Wang Y, et al. Predictors of readmission among elderly survivors of admission with heart failure. Am Heart J 2000;139(1 I):72–7.

129. Arundel C, Lam PH, Khosla R, et al. Association of 30-day all-cause readmission with long-term outcomes in hospitalized older medicare beneficiaries with heart failure. Am J Med 2016;129(11): 1178–84.

130. Greene SJ, Butler J, Albert NM, et al. Medical therapy for heart failure with reduced ejection fraction: the CHAMP-HF registry. J Am Coll Cardiol 2018; 72(4):351–66.

131. Greene SJ, Fonarow GC, DeVore AD, et al. Titration of medical therapy for heart failure with reduced ejection fraction. J Am Coll Cardiol 2019;73(19): 2365–83.

132. Roth GA, Poole JE, Zaha R, et al. Use of guideline-directed medications for heart failure before cardioverter-defibrillator implantation. J Am Coll Cardiol 2016;67(9):1062–9.

133. Joynt Maddox KE, Reidhead M, Hu J, et al. Adjusting for social risk factors impacts performance and penalties in the hospital readmissions reduction program. Health Serv Res 2019;54(2): 327–36.

134. Meddings J, Reichert H, Smith SN, et al. The impact of disability and social determinants of health on condition-specific readmissions beyond medicare risk adjustments: a cohort study. J Gen Intern Med 2017;32(1):71–80.

135. Foraker RE, Rose KM, Suchindran CM, et al. Socioeconomic status, medicaid coverage, clinical comorbidity, and rehospitalization or death after an incident heart failure hospitalization atherosclerosis risk in communities cohort (1987 to 2004). Circ Heart Fail 2011;4(3):308–16.

136. Bikdeli B, Wayda B, Bao H, et al. Place of residence and outcomes of patients with heart failure: Analysis from the telemonitoring to improve heart failure outcomes trial. Circ Cardiovasc Qual Outcomes 2014;7(5):749–56.

137. Lee DS, Austin PC, Rouleau JL, et al. Predicting mortality among patients hospitalized for heart failure: derivation and validation of a clinical model. J Am Med Assoc 2003;290(19):2581–7.

138. Loghmanpour NA, Kormos RL, Kanwar MK, et al. A Bayesian model to predict right ventricular failure following left ventricular assist device therapy. JACC Hear Fail 2016;4(9):711–21.

139. Mortazavi BJ, Downing NS, Bucholz EM, et al. Analysis of machine learning techniques for heart failure readmissions. Circ Cardiovasc Qual Outcomes 2016;9(6):629–40.

140. Frizzell JD, Liang L, Schulte PJ, et al. Prediction of 30-day all-cause readmissions in patients hospitalized for heart failure: Comparison of machine learning and other statistical approaches. JAMA Cardiol 2017;2(2):204–9.

141. Ahmad T, Lund LH, Rao P, et al. Machine learning methods improve prognostication, identify clinically distinct phenotypes, and detect heterogeneity in response to therapy in a large cohort of heart

failure patients. J Am Heart Assoc 2018;7(8). https://doi.org/10.1161/JAHA.117.008081.

142. Golas SB, Shibahara T, Agboola S, et al. A machine learning model to predict the risk of 30-day readmissions in patients with heart failure: A retrospective analysis of electronic medical records data. BMC Med Inform Decis Mak 2018;18(1). https://doi.org/10.1186/s12911-018-0620-z.

143. Adler ED, Voors AA, Klein L, et al. Improving risk prediction in heart failure using machine learning. Eur J Heart Fail 2019;1–9. https://doi.org/10.1002/ejhf.1628.

144. Angraal S, Mortazavi BJ, Gupta A, et al. Machine Learning Prediction of Mortality and Hospitalization in Heart Failure with Preserved Ejection Fraction. JACC Hear Fail 2019;8(1). https://doi.org/10.1016/j.jchf.2019.06.013.

145. Desai RJ, Wang SV, Vaduganathan M, et al. Comparison of machine learning methods with traditional models for use of administrative claims with electronic medical records to predict heart failure outcomes. JAMA Netw Open 2020;3(1): 1–15.

Empowering People Living with Heart Failure

Peter Wohlfahrt, MD, PhD[a,b,c], Josef Stehlik, MD, MPH[a], Irene Z. Pan, PharmD[d,e], John J. Ryan, MD, MB BCh, BAO[a,*]

KEYWORDS

- Cardiomyopathy • Pulmonary hypertension • Patient-reported outcomes
- Remote patient monitoring • Dyspnea • Pharmacists • Patient-centered medical homes

KEY POINTS

- Empowering patients is a proactive process that involves patients' self-efficacy and capacity to make informed decisions about their health care. Heart failure is a chronic disease in which patient activation and empowering are particularly valuable.
- Patient empowerment requires attention and dedication to the reevaluation and reimagination of the framework providers currently use to deliver care.
- As patients seek to take on a more active role in the management of their disease state, integration of a pharmacist onto a multidisciplinary team can increase patient understanding of their medical regimen and therefore their ability to make informed decisions regarding their care.
- Physicians often fail to recognize functional disabilities reported by their patients. Standardized, valid, reproducible, and sensitive patient-reported outcomes that capture patients' experience with their illness may be needed to overcome this limitation.

INTRODUCTION

The continued increase in health care expenditures has incentivized a search for an improved, value-driven health care delivery model. Patient-centeredness has been identified as one of the essential pillars of a value-driven approach aimed at improvement in the quality of health care.[1] In patient-centered care, patients' specific health needs and desired health outcomes are the driving force behind all health care decisions. Patient-centered care requires active involvement of patients in their treatment, whereby the traditional passive role of a patient as a recipient of care is replaced by a relationship in which the patient takes an equal and active role. Thus, the patient becomes both a partner with the provider and an important resource in decision making. The person cannot become lost in the patient. For this reason, the authors think the emphasis should be on empowering *people* living with heart failure (HF), not just patients. This transformation of the patient's role is facilitated by recent technological advances, which include better access to information through Internet and social media and advances in remote monitoring and artificial intelligence. However, in order for the implementation of a patient-centered model to be effective,

Funding: Dr J.J. Ryan and his research are supported by funding from The Reagan Corporation, The Gordon Family, and The Cushman Family. Dr Stehlik's and Dr Wohlfahrt's work was supported by the American Heart Association HF SFRN grant 16SFRN31890003 (PI: Stehlik J). Dr Wohlfahrt's work was supported by a research grant awarded by Ministry of Health of the Czech Republic, grant nr. NV 19-09-00125.

[a] Division of Cardiovascular Medicine, Department of Medicine, University of Utah, Salt Lake City, Utah, USA; [b] Center for Cardiovascular Prevention, Charles University in Prague, First Faculty of Medicine and Thomayer Hospital, Prague, Czech Republic; [c] Department of Preventive Cardiology, Institute for Clinical and Experimental Medicine, Prague, Czech Republic; [d] Department of Pharmacy, University of Utah Health, Salt Lake City, Utah, USA; [e] College of Pharmacy, University of Utah, Salt Lake City, Utah, USA
* Corresponding author. University of Utah Health Science Center, 30 North 1900 East, Room 4A100, Salt Lake City, UT 84132.
E-mail address: john.ryan@hsc.utah.edu

Heart Failure Clin 16 (2020) 409–420
https://doi.org/10.1016/j.hfc.2020.06.002

one must reconfigure the patient-provider relationship (**Fig. 1**). As previously noted, "the doctors need to come down off the pedestal and the patients have to get up off their knees."[2]

Activation and empowerment of people with chronic illness can be viewed as a hierarchical process that includes people accumulating knowledge, confidence, and self-determination for their own health care.[3] Although patient activation refers to patients' knowledge, skill, and confidence to manage their health and health care,[4] empowering patients is a more proactive process, which involves patients' self-efficacy and capacity to make informed decisions about their health care.[5] Patient activation is required for their empowering. An informed person is more likely to develop confidence.[6] With confidence, people can be motivated and gain self-determination abilities, such as the ability to efficiently communicate with their providers, and express their health concerns and preferences. Self-determination empowers people to seek more health information, acquire more knowledge of their health from providers or other sources, and become more confident.

In several areas of medicine, patient activation and empowering have been shown to be effective in improving medical outcomes and lowering health care costs. For example, self-management of oral anticoagulation among people with atrial fibrillation has been used by select centers with some success rather than relying exclusively on clinic-based management of anticoagulation.[7] Another example of effective patient

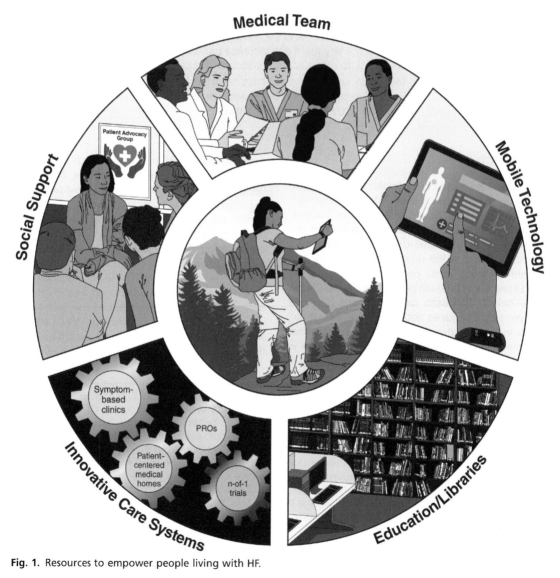

Fig. 1. Resources to empower people living with HF.

empowering is self-monitoring of blood glucose in patients with diabetes mellitus.[8,9]

HF is a chronic disease associated with significant disability, in which patient activation and empowering are particularly valuable. Patient involvement allows providers to understand which outcomes are most valued by the person living with HF, which in turn can have a direct impact on therapy selection. Knowing patient's preferences is particularly relevant for therapies that provide symptom relief, but have not been shown to improve survival (eg, chronic intravenous inotropes), and in decisions regarding selection for advanced HF therapies, including heart transplant or left ventricular assist device support. Another aspect whereby patient activation and empowering could impact outcomes is mitigation of the risk of hospitalization, an event responsible for 80% of HF health care cost. However, more research is needed to determine how to best translate patient activation, empowering self-care.[10]

In this review, the authors discuss practical approaches to activate and empower people with HF and enable patient-provider dialogue and shared decision making.

PATIENT EMPOWERMENT

Patient empowerment first requires them to be recognized by themselves as well as by their providers as people not patients. Identifying people rather than patients removes much of the hierarchy of health care delivery and reminds all involved of the shared responsibility and immense possibility of shared decision making when viewed as partners in health care, not just subservient patients, relying on instruction from clinicians. Empowering people living with HF requires establishing guidelines and giving direction as to what aspects of their health and their care they should take charge of. The extent to which people can take charge in their care depends on their level of comfort and the shared confidence of the patient, their provider, and their family. As part of empowerment, people living with HF can monitor their symptoms; adhere to their medication regimen; and design and follow through with diet and exercise routines. In addition to recognizing changes in their symptoms, people with HF can also take charge of responding to these changes by either seeking assistance from their providers or adapting their own behavior and medications through pre-agreed-upon protocols. Self-management is integral to achieving the best outcomes in HF.[11] In fact, self-management has been shown to be associated with fewer hospital admissions, improved quality of life (QoL), and decreased mortality, in particular, as it pertains to changes in medication. What is less clear is the exact impact and the best way to optimize changes in lifestyle and fluid intake.[12]

As part of self-management and patient empowerment, people with HF may need to learn new skills, such as how to monitor and manage symptoms and complex medication regimens. People may also need to adapt and maintain other behaviors, such as exercise regularly, stop smoking and restrict fluid and sodium intake. However, targets such as restricting fluid intake and reporting weight gains if greater than 5 pounds (or >2 kg) over 3 days need to be individualized according to symptoms, disease state, and personal expectations. Although such individualization increases the complexity and the demands of self-care, this sense of control and achievement also increases the empowerment from taking charge of one's health. This self-care also requires flexibility on the part of the provider, because, for example, diuretic dosing may need to be individualized to suit the lifestyle, habits, and social calendar of the patient, rather than relying simply on "best practice" or standard recommended timing and schedule from the prescriber. Self-care and patient empowerment require a partnership with and mutual confidence between the health care team and the patient. In order to safely and successfully have individuals manage their own diuretic doses, the parameters and targets, especially weight, need to be regularly reviewed at clinic visits. Resetting target weights is important and difficult to do. Doing so requires evaluating jugular venous distension, blood pressure, symptoms, as well as brain-natriuretic peptide level and kidney function. Upon completion of this evaluation, providers and patients can then agree on what the new target weight will be and then revisit on subsequent visits.

One of the challenges to self-management is level of health literacy.[13] Poor health literacy may contribute to poor clinical outcomes either directly or secondary to low socioeconomic status, poor access to health care, and poor relationships between health care providers and patients. Therefore, in order to improve self-care, health care literacy will also need to be improved. Limitations, such as decreased overall literacy levels, physical or cognitive impairment, and co-morbidities, including depression and anxiety, need to be addressed because they can undermine the ability to participate in self-management. Depression and anxiety in particular are associated with poor adherence to medical regimens. Therefore, aggressively managing depression is important in order for people to become engaged in their self-care. In addition, consistency in the construct of the care team, comprising doctors, advanced practice clinicians, clinical pharmacists, and social workers, among others, helps ensure continuity of effort in promoting self-management as well as provides patients with familiarity, which in turn can ease anxiety surrounding the extra responsibilities provided to them.

Specialized programs have been introduced to encourage patient empowerment and address the complex nature of individualized care in HF. Studies looking at these programs have shown mixed or oftentimes neutral results. The HART trial targeted patient willingness and capacity to self-care through counseling and group education to optimize "*self-monitoring, environmental restructuring, elicitation of support from family and friends, cognitive restructuring and the relaxation response.*"[14] More than 900 patients were randomized to education alone (enhanced standard care) or to an education and counseling program. Of note, after 12 months, there was no difference in mortality or hospital readmission in the education-alone group compared with the self-management group. A study of 93 patients by Shao and colleagues[15] showed that people with HF who were randomized to a 12-week nurse-led self-management program showed significantly better symptom control and management than usual care patients. The self-management program emphasized patient control of sodium and fluid intake. In a similar 6-week nurse-led program in 317 patients by Smeulders and colleagues,[16] significant effects were found for cognitive symptom management, self-care, and QoL. However, these effects were not sustained at 6- or 12-month follow-up.

Social Networks and Patient Advocacy Groups

Rather than putting an emphasis on self-care, it is perhaps worth considering if a preferable approach would be to rely on peer-support programs to target a phrase the authors are coining called *collective-care*, whereby the group at large, comprising others with HF, work together and share best practices so that the group as a whole sees an improvement in their health. Peer-support programs have been shown to improve patient self-management in some chronic diseases, such as type 2 diabetes mellitus.[17] Social networks have already been shown to change the needs and expectations of patients with heart disease,[18] and it stands to reason that they would have a similar effect in HF. Poor engagement in self-care

programs may be overcome by strategies offered over social networks, which provide opportunities to integrate care into the existing platforms for connectivity. These social networks therefore do not necessarily have to be in person but rather can be through online platforms. In turn, these social networks oftentimes are seen partnering up or connecting with patient advocacy groups, which are very active in disease states, such as amyloidosis and hypertrophic cardiomyopathy. These patient advocacy groups can empower people with HF, especially those with less common forms of heart failure, by increasing awareness of clinical trials, centers of excellence, new therapies, and patient-assistance programs.

REIMAGINING CLINICAL CARE
Symptom-Based Clinics

Patient empowerment requires attention and dedication to the reevaluation and reimagination of the framework providers currently use to deliver care. As it stands, specialized areas of clinical care are oftentimes further divided into subspecialties. Within cardiology, patients are directed to specialists siloed to the part of the heart affected, for instance, valve clinic, HF clinic, heart rhythm clinic, or even pulmonary hypertension clinic. This care model is largely organized around the physician specialist. However, on initial presentation, patients rarely, if ever, distinctly complain, "I have a valve problem," or "I have pulmonary hypertension." Rather, they present with subjective symptoms, such as shortness of breath, palpitations, or angina. The pathologic condition attributed to those symptoms is subsequently identified, and these patients are referred on to the respective clinic. However, the world of medicine is very rarely black and white, and signs and symptoms often overlap between disease states. In order to empower patients, it is worth reexamining and potentially restructuring the current model. One such approach that has begun to take root is the introduction of clinics revolving around symptoms rather than a particular disease state. Through this model, the patient's complaints are at the front and center of their clinic visit, and in doing so, this becomes the primary target of care delivery. A prime example of this evolving model is the dyspnea clinic, where patients with unexplained shortness of breath are referred for evaluation.[19] Such clinics are growing in popularity, particularly in North America. Patients complaining of dyspnea can bounce between specialists for upwards of 2 years before receiving a diagnosis.[20] The time and expense for the evaluation of dyspnea can be significant and oftentimes can lead to duplicate workup and testing. For these reasons, practice settings, such as dyspnea clinics, headache clinics, faint and fall clinics, and others, can provide a more targeted approach in which the patient's symptoms are placed at the forefront of the clinical evaluation.[19,21] This emphasis on what brought the patient into the doctor's office in the first place serves to inform and to guide the conversation between the provider and the patient. Framing their symptoms and functional status in the context of the pathologic condition of their disease encourages patients to take an active role in their care and helps to facilitate treatment plans that target patient-specific goals with the guidance of their health care provider.

Clinical Trials

Clinical trials have the potential to engage patients more within their care, especially for patients with HF with preserved ejection fraction, whereby treatment options are very limited. By being a part of something greater than oneself, patients can feel empowered and excited to contribute to the medical literature. The traditional randomized controlled trial remains the backbone of clinical research, but novel trial designs are being used to provide people living with HF more options. One such novel trial design is the n-of-1 clinical trial, which the authors detail more in later discussion.

N-of-1 Studies

When developing a clinical care plan in conjunction with a patient, the clinician may be faced with treatment strategies that lack strong clinical data support. In particular, although an increasing number of new therapies have been shown to provide benefit in systolic HF,[22–24] patients with right HF do not have the same options. Therefore, another mechanism with which clinicians may empower patients is to propose an n-of-1 clinical trial, whereby the patient leads and participates in a clinical trial of a therapeutic agent or strategy.[25] Before the start of the trial, the patient and the care team decide on the study parameters and determine what will define success or failure of an intervention. After a prespecified period of time, the patient and the providers review the patient's progress and elect whether to continue or discontinue the intervention.

An example worth considering is a patient presenting with pulmonary arterial hypertension (PAH), or group 1 PH, with risk factors for pulmonary hypertension secondary to left-sided heart disease, or group 2 PH. There are currently no Food and Drug Administration (FDA)-approved therapies for group 2 PH. In the setting of a patient with multiple risk factors for various groups of pulmonary hypertension, it is reasonable to consider performing an n-of-1 clinical trial with a PAH-specific therapy in order to uncover potential clinical response. The patient and the provider select objective measurements, such as 6-minute walk test, distinctive features on echocardiogram, and brain natriuretic peptide level. These measurements are taken at baseline and repeated at 12 weeks from when the PAH-specific therapy is first introduced. The objective and subjective data are reviewed in the context of prespecified measures of success, as determined by the patient. If improved, the patient and the care team may elect to continue the therapy. However, if these parameters have worsened or the patient's functional status has declined, the patient and providers have already committed to discontinuing the medication. These trials can be formalized through institutional review boards, or they can be contractual in the clinical setting. Most importantly, such trials require the patient to define ahead of time what success will look like to them and empower them to be the judge of that success (or failure).

Patient-Centered Medical Home

Another method to empower patients living with HF is the creation of a patient-centered medical home (PCMH). HF patients are often treated by a revolving door of providers, including primary care, cardiologists, sleep specialists, pharmacists, social workers, physical therapists, and more. This model promotes an integrated environment that fosters comprehensive, patient-centered, and team-based care with a focus on quality and safety. Although well established in primary care, PCMHs have not yet become a recognized model in the management of HF. The medical home comprises of a team of care providers, who are accountable for a patient's physical and mental health care needs, including wellness and prevention, acute care, and chronic care. Care is organized across all elements of the broader health care system, including specialty care, hospitals, home health care, and community services. A partnership is developed and cultivated between the practitioners, the patients, and their families (if appropriate) to ensure clinical decision making respects the patients' goals and preferences. In addition, this partnership ensures the infrastructure is put into place so that patients have the education and support they need to make decisions and participate in their own care. This model, when done properly, empowers the patient by placing them at the center of their care and would be a reasonable offering in HF clinics.[26–28]

Utilization of Clinical Pharmacists

HF, and in particular, HF with reduced ejection fraction, is a disease managed in large part with pharmacologic therapies, including but not limited to beta-blockers, angiotensin receptor-neprilysn inhibitors/angiotensin converting enzyme inhibitors/angiotensin receptor blockers, aldosterone receptor antagonists, loop diuretics, and most recently, sodium-glucose cotransporter-2 inhibitors.[23,29] Given the complexity of medication management in HF (and other common comorbidities seen in HF patients), the incorporation of a trained clinical pharmacist in both the inpatient and the outpatient settings can have a large impact on medication adherence, patient knowledge of disease state, overall patient satisfaction, and hospital readmission rates.[30] In addition, as an increasing number of pharmacologic treatments become available, pharmacists are in a unique position to educate providers and patients on drug treatment, monitor for potential adverse reactions or drug-drug interactions, and tailor drug regimens to individual patients for effectiveness, tolerability, cost, and patient goals of care.

As patients seek to take on a more active role in the management of their disease state, integration of a pharmacist onto a multidisciplinary team can increase patient understanding of their medical regimen and therefore their ability to make informed decisions regarding their care. One example of shared decision making in HF focuses on having the patient and the clinical team establish medication titration protocols to address hypervolemia. The incorporation of a trained clinical pharmacist has been shown to improve optimization of HF medications and decrease the likelihood of adverse events, such as renal impairment or hyperkalemia.[31,32]

Group visits

A group visit is an interactive, scheduled group appointment with a heart care provider and a small number of patients who share a medical condition. The process of the group visit can vary, but typically it involves 6 to 12 patients gathered together for 1 to 2 hours to discuss education and health concerns. They have been shown to be successful in hypertension, diabetes, and other chronic diseases. Group visits have also been studied in HF and can be used to optimize medication therapy while providing a forum for knowledge acquisition

and fostering support.[33] These benefits are clearly consistent with the goal of patient empowerment. Depending on the goal of each group visit, it can be run by different health care professionals. For example, a group visit in HF focused on nutrition and healthy eating may best be run by a registered dietician. Similarly, if the goal of the group visit is to provide insight and recommendations regarding exercise and activity, then exercise physiologists or physical therapists may be able to run that visit. It is important to set expectations for those in attendance before the group visit, so that patients and their caregivers can come with questions and defined goals.

PATIENT-REPORTED OUTCOMES

Physician understanding of patient health status, goals, and values is essential in HF management and decision making.[34] Traditionally, providers have relied on fairly unstructured patient questioning to determine symptom burden and QoL. However, this approach is time demanding and influenced by provider skills and subjective interpretation.[35] Furthermore, physicians often fail to recognize functional disabilities reported by their patients.[36] Thus, standardized, valid, reproducible, and sensitive instruments that capture patients' experience with their illness may be needed to overcome this limitation. Patient-reported outcomes (PROs) can be particularly helpful in this goal.

PROs are defined as reports coming directly from patients about how they feel or function in relation to a health condition and its therapy, without interpretation by health care providers or anyone else.[37] PROs can provide HF-specific information or can evaluate general health-related QoL. Although HF-specific instruments measure QoL domains relevant to HF, general QoL instruments assess overall well-being and integrate the influence of HF and other comorbidities on QoL. For clinical practice, a combination of HF-specific and generic instruments may be valuable.

Heart Failure-Specific Patient-Reported Outcomes Instruments

Although several HF-specific PRO tools have been developed, the Kansas City Cardiomyopathy Questionnaire (KCCQ) and the Minnesota Living with Heart Failure Questionnaire (MLHFQ) are 2 instruments that fulfill all criteria deemed important for clinical use, which include content and construct validity, reliability, responsiveness, performance diversity, feasibility, interpretability, and prognostic value.[34,38]

Minnesota Living with Heart Failure Questionnaire

The MLHFQ has 21 items, which can be completed in less than 10 minutes. It provides information on physical, emotional, and social dimension of QoL impairment and a total score.[39] Although the MLHFQ has good responsiveness to clinical status improvement in patients with HF, including HF with preserved ejection fraction,[40] it does not reflect well clinical status deterioration.[41,42] This observation is also supported by a study among patients discharged for HF exacerbation, in which improvement in MLHFQ (defined as a total score decrease of more than 5 points) was associated with better rehospitalization-free survival, whereas there was no significant difference in the outcome between those with no change and MLHFQ score worsening.[43]

Kansas City Cardiomyopathy Questionnaire

The 23 item KCCQ questionnaire includes physical limitation, HF symptoms stability, burden and frequency, self-efficacy, QoL, and social limitation domains and requires 5 to 8 minutes to complete.[44] Two summary scores are also calculated: the global summary score, which includes all domains, and the clinical summary score, which includes only the physical limitation and symptoms domains. The summary scores range from 0 to 100, with scores less than 25 marking very severe HF-related QoL impairment, whereas a score greater than 75 is associated with very good to excellent QoL.[45] KCCQ score is sensitive to clinical changes, with a 5-point change over follow-up marking clinically significant change in HF status.[46] Furthermore, a 5-point change in KCCQ score is associated with an 11% change in the hazard ratio of hospitalization and cardiovascular death.[47] A clinically significant worsening of the global KCCQ score requires a closer look at each of KCCQ domains to determine if the patient needs adjustment in HF medication or other invasive intervention, or to involve therapist, counselor, or palliative care if QoL has deteriorated in the absence of a change in symptoms or functional limitations. More recently, a short 12-item version of KCCQ has been introduced, which requires only 2 to 3 minutes for completion, and retains all psychometric properties of the full KCCQ.[48]

Generic Patient-Reported Outcomes Instruments

Because patients with HF have multiple comorbidities, it may be difficult to attribute symptoms to a single condition. Generic PROs integrate the influence of multiple health conditions on QoL. Among patients with HF, the PROMIS and VAS instruments may be particularly valuable.

Patient-reported outcome information system

PROMIS is a publicly available system of person-centered measures that evaluates and monitors physical, mental, and social health. Measures were developed for children and adults and have been translated into greater than 40 languages. The PROMIS bank has 70 domains, of which physical function, fatigue, depression, and satisfaction with social roles may be relevant to HF. PROMIS uses computerized adaptive testing, which increases the precision of assessment, while decreasing respondent burden. The PROMIS score ranges from 0 to 100 with higher scores indicating a higher level of the symptom measured, for example, more fatigue and better physical function.

Visual analogue scale

The State of Health Visual analogue scale (VAS; a component of the EuroQoL 5 Dimensions) is a generic QoL instrument that records the respondent's self-rated perception of health status. The VAS score ranges from 0 to 100, with the score 0 labeled "Worst imaginable health state" and the score 100 labeled "Best imaginable health state." The patient is instructed to simply "mark an X on the scale" to indicate how their health is on the day of the assessment. This information can be used as a quantitative measure of health outcome as judged by the individual respondent.

Benefit of Patient-Reported Outcomes Use in Clinical Care of Heart Failure Patients

PROs have been routinely used in clinical trials of HF therapies to determine the effect of the studied interventions on patient QoL. More recently, use of PROs in routine clinical care has been examined.[49] The potential benefits of PRO implementation in HF clinical practice are summarized in **Table 1**.

Patient-Reported Outcomes Implementation in Heart Failure

Despite the apparent advantages of routine use of PROs, their introduction into clinical care has been limited. In **Table 2**, the authors provide recommendations for PRO implementation in HF. In particular, emphasis on provider education, seamless data collection and scoring, interpretable presentation of results, and selection of relevant and actionable PROs are important aspects that will facilitate successful implementation of PROs into clinical practice. Although it is generally assumed that PRO use in clinical practice will improve care, the impact of routine PRO use on outcomes

Table 1
Benefit of patient-reported outcomes implementation

Benefit	Comments
Identify disconnect between patient and provider perspective on symptoms, function, and QoL	• Physicians underestimate or fail to recognize functional disabilities that are reported by their patients[36]
Reproducibility	• Relevant questions asked in the same way each time • Eliminate provider variability in QoL assessment
Sensitivity to change	• Can detect change in HF-related QoL and the impact of therapy[41,46]
Time-efficient	• Self-administered • Can replace unstructured questioning on functional status • Can be repeated as frequently • Reproducible results obtained within minutes
Access to health care	• PRO instruments available in many languages • Facilitate intervention planning
Prognostic information	• Prediction of survival and hospitalization[45,47,65]

has not been well established. Randomized trials are needed to assess the additive value of routine use of PROs in clinical practice on outcomes, including mortality, rehospitalization, health status, and satisfaction with care.

REMOTE PATIENT MONITORING

Recent advances in wireless communication and biomedical sensors represent another development that is shifting the health care delivery from a clinic-centric to a patient-centric model. Remote patient monitoring (RPM) seeks to use patient information obtained outside of the health care setting to better manage their chronic conditions.[50] Remote monitoring uses patient-generated data that are transferred to a health care team and are used to tailor therapy by providers or by the patients themselves. In order to avoid provider data overflow, an automated analytical process (eg, artificial intelligence) may be used to flag and alert abnormal actionable readings.

RPM technology can empower patients by giving them more control over their health and treatment and by improving self-management. For HF providers, RPM can be used to evaluate patient's adherence to a treatment, detect early changes in clinical status, and plan intervention before a costly care episode occurs. The promise of RPM in HF is a decrease in the risk of rehospitalization, better QoL, better survival, and improved access to specialized care for patients at risk. The field is rapidly evolving, and the optimal and efficient ways of RPM integration into HF care are still to be identified.

Noninvasive Remote Patient Monitoring

There is conflicting evidence on the utility of noninvasive RPM in HF. Although small-scale and single-center trials demonstrated benefit,[51] 5 large prospective randomized trials failed to show benefit of RPM compared with standard care.[52–56] Potential explanations for the lack of RPM benefit include poor adherence of patients to remote monitoring and failure to take action in response to a clinical alert triggered by the information obtained through RPM, implying that higher patient engagement and better implementation of the tested approaches into clinical workflow need to be pursued. RPM technology with focus on user-centered design is likely to appeal to patients of a wide range of age, health, and digital literacy and may improve adherence to the intervention.[57] Furthermore, patient selection may also play an important role in the efficacy of RPM, such as use during times of elevated risk, for example, after discharge for HF exacerbation.

Invasive Remote Patient Monitoring

Utility of several implantable devices to detect impeding HF exacerbation and to decrease HF hospitalizations has been tested. Several studies examined measurement of intrathoracic impedance using implantable cardioverter-defibrillators or cardiac resynchronization therapy. An analytical algorithm was applied to serial thoracic impedance measurements over time to identify patients

Table 2
Recommendations for patient-reported outcomes implementation in heart failure

Barrier	Recommendation
Data collection	
Burden	Secure administrative and financial support
	Achieve full engagement of the providers and patients
	Optimize workflow
	• Replace unstructured questioning on functional status with PROs
	• Assess PROs before the clinic visit, ideally through online data submission
	• Use real-time scoring of PROs with electronic health record integration
	• PROs frequency: HF-specific PROs with every encounter, comprehensive PRO panel at 3- to 6-mo intervals
Language and health literacy/cognitive barriers	Use available PRO instrument translations
	Patient proxy or a nurse may assist in completing PROs
Results presentation	Present PRO trends with time on the x-axis and the PRO score on the y-axis
Ambiguous meaning of scales	Educate providers on PRO interpretation
Summary score vs domain score	Provide summary score with the option to review domain scores
PRO utility and clinical value	
Clinical judgment supersedes PRO	Educate providers on PRO nature, utility, and additional value over standard history taking
Actionable PRO data	Educate providers on PRO thresholds for action
	More research needed on the advantages of treatment decisions/shared decision making integrating PRO results
PROs selection	Implement both HF-specific and generic PROs in HF clinics
	Prevent repeating the same or similar questions when combining multiple PROs
Intended audience for PROs	Approach all providers that participate in the care of HF patients

at risk for HF exacerbation.[58] However, the predictive accuracy to detect impeding HF varied considerably among studies, ranging from 21% to 76%,[59–61] and this approach based on only 1 parameter was negatively affected by frequent false alarms. In a more recent approach, data from multiple sensors are analyzed. The Multi-SENSE study described an algorithm based on several variables collected from a cardiac resynchronization therapy device/implantable defibrillator that had 70% sensitivity for detection of subsequent hospitalization or outpatient visit for worsening of HF.[62] Whether this approach leads to A clinically meaningful decrease in HF hospitalization and QoL improvement needs further evaluation.

In the only randomized study to date that has shown reduction of hospitalization compared with standard care, data from implantable pulmonary artery pressure monitor CardioMEMS (Abbott Laboratoris, Atlanta, Georgia, USA) were used by HF providers to make adjustments to medical therapy. This device has been approved by the FDA for clinical use.[63,64] Additional studies determining optimal use of the data and studies to define cost-effectiveness of the system are needed.

Future Direction of Remote Patient Monitoring in Heart Failure

Multiple implantable and wearable monitors designed to notify providers of the risk of HF exacerbation have been developed or are under development. Although some of these devices have been shown to predict the risk of HF hospitalization, future studies need to test how to best implement this technology-based approach into clinical practice. A critical step in achieving clinical efficacy will be to ensure high levels of adoption and acceptability in clinical settings with careful attention to workflow, implementation fidelity, and patient experience. Closed-loop decision pathways that minimize the need for provider decision making could increase the response rate to alerts. Similarly, better engagement could be achieved through sharing of the results with patients and through involvement of patients in decision making regarding treatment modifications prompted by RPM.

SUMMARY

The increased resources available for HF provide people more options, more awareness, and more understanding of their disease. It is hoped that this contributes to people living with HF to feeling more empowered (see **Fig. 1**). However, it does require a partnership with their clinical team in order to ensure that the modern technologies and the self-care that comes with empowerment are being used in a positive, effective way. Over time, best practices in empowering people living with HF will be developed, and a continued effort to improve the patient experience will require close partnership between those living with HF and those caring for HF.

ACKNOWLEDGMENTS

The authors thank Patrick Lane, www. sceyencestudios.com, for his work on the figure.

DISCLOSURE

The authors have nothing to disclose.

REFERENCES

1. Institute of Medicine Committee on Quality of Health Care in A. Crossing the quality chasm: a new health system for the 21st century. Washington (DC): National Academies Press (US); 2001.
2. Kane J. How doctors and patients can heal our sick system. New York: Helios Press; 2015.
3. Chen J, Mullins CD, Novak P, et al. Personalized strategies to activate and empower patients in health care and reduce health disparities. Health Educ Behav 2016;43(1):25–34.
4. Hibbard JH, Greene J. What the evidence shows about patient activation: better health outcomes and care experiences; fewer data on costs. Health Aff (Millwood) 2013;32(2):207–14.
5. Aujoulat I, Marcolongo R, Bonadiman L, et al. Reconsidering patient empowerment in chronic illness: a critique of models of self-efficacy and bodily control. Soc Sci Med 2008;66(5):1228–39.
6. Ludman EJ, Peterson D, Katon WJ, et al. Improving confidence for self care in patients with depression and chronic illnesses. Behav Med 2013;39(1):1–6.
7. Heneghan CJ, Garcia-Alamino JM, Spencer EA, et al. Self-monitoring and self-management of oral anticoagulation. Cochrane Database Syst Rev 2016;(7):CD003839.
8. Guerci B, Drouin P, Grange V, et al. Self-monitoring of blood glucose significantly improves metabolic control in patients with type 2 diabetes mellitus: the Auto-Surveillance Intervention Active (ASIA) study. Diabetes Metab 2003;29(6):587–94.
9. Barnett AH, Krentz AJ, Strojek K, et al. The efficacy of self-monitoring of blood glucose in the management of patients with type 2 diabetes treated with a gliclazide modified release-based regimen. A multicentre, randomized, parallel-group, 6-month evaluation (DINAMIC 1 study). Diabetes Obes Metab 2008;10(12):1239–47.
10. Grady KL. Self-care and quality of life outcomes in heart failure patients. J Cardiovasc Nurs 2008;23(3):285–92.
11. McMurray JJ, Adamopoulos S, Anker SD, et al. ESC Guidelines for the diagnosis and treatment of acute and chronic heart failure 2012: the Task Force for the Diagnosis and Treatment of Acute and Chronic Heart Failure 2012 of the European Society of Cardiology. Developed in collaboration with the Heart Failure Association (HFA) of the ESC. Eur Heart J 2012;33(14):1787–847.
12. Lainscak M, Blue L, Clark AL, et al. Self-care management of heart failure: practical recommendations from the Patient Care Committee of the Heart Failure Association of the European Society of Cardiology. Eur J Heart Fail 2011;13(2):115–26.
13. van der Wal MH, Jaarsma T, Moser DK, et al. Compliance in heart failure patients: the importance of knowledge and beliefs. Eur Heart J 2006;27(4):434–40.
14. Powell LH, Calvin JE Jr, Richardson D, et al. Self-management counseling in patients with heart failure: the heart failure adherence and retention randomized behavioral trial. JAMA 2010;304(12):1331–8.
15. Shao JH, Chang AM, Edwards H, et al. A randomized controlled trial of self-management programme improves health-related outcomes of older people with heart failure. J Adv Nurs 2013;69(11):2458–69.
16. Smeulders ES, van Haastregt JC, Ambergen T, et al. Nurse-led self-management group programme for patients with congestive heart failure: randomized controlled trial. J Adv Nurs 2010;66(7):1487–99.
17. Trento M, Gamba S, Gentile L, et al. Rethink Organization to iMprove Education and Outcomes (ROMEO): a multicenter randomized trial of lifestyle intervention by group care to manage type 2 diabetes. Diabetes Care 2010;33(4):745–7.

18. Reeves D, Blickem C, Vassilev I, et al. The contribution of social networks to the health and self-management of patients with long-term conditions: a longitudinal study. PLoS One 2014;9(6):e98340.

19. Ryan JJ, Waxman AB. The dyspnea clinic. Circulation 2018;137(19):1994–6.

20. Huang W, Resch S, Oliveira RK, et al. Invasive cardiopulmonary exercise testing in the evaluation of unexplained dyspnea: insights from a multidisciplinary dyspnea center. Eur J Prev Cardiol 2017; 24(11):1190–9.

21. Sanders NA, Jetter TL, Brignole M, et al. Standardized care pathway versus conventional approach in the management of patients presenting with faint at the University of Utah. Pacing Clin Electrophysiol 2013;36(2):152–62.

22. McMurray JJ, Packer M, Desai AS, et al. Angiotensin-neprilysin inhibition versus enalapril in heart failure. N Engl J Med 2014;371(11):993–1004.

23. McMurray JJV, Solomon SD, Inzucchi SE, et al. Dapagliflozin in patients with heart failure and reduced ejection fraction. N Engl J Med 2019;381(21): 1995–2008.

24. Armstrong PW, Roessig L, Patel MJ, et al. A multicenter, randomized, double-blind, placebo-controlled trial of the efficacy and safety of the oral soluble guanylate cyclase stimulator: the VICTORIA Trial. JACC Heart Fail 2018;6(2):96–104.

25. Ryan JJ, Rich JD, Maron BA. Building the case for novel clinical trials in pulmonary arterial hypertension. Circ Cardiovasc Qual Outcomes 2015;8(1): 114–23.

26. Arend J, Tsang-Quinn J, Levine C, et al. The patient-centered medical home: history, components, and review of the evidence. Mt Sinai J Med 2012;79(4): 433–50.

27. Shi L, Lee DC, Chung M, et al. Patient-centered medical home recognition and clinical performance in U.S. community health centers. Health Serv Res 2017;52(3):984–1004.

28. Fernandes SM, Sanders LM. Patient-centered medical home for patients with complex congenital heart disease. Curr Opin Pediatr 2015;27(5): 581–6.

29. Yancy CW, Jessup M, Bozkurt B, et al. 2017 ACC/AHA/HFSA focused update of the 2013 ACCF/AHA Guideline for the Management of Heart Failure: a report of the American College of Cardiology/American Heart Association Task Force on Clinical Practice Guidelines and the Heart Failure Society of America. Circulation 2017;136(6):e137–61.

30. Parajuli DR, Franzon J, McKinnon RA, et al. Role of the pharmacist for improving self-care and outcomes in heart failure. Curr Heart Fail Rep 2017; 14(2):78–86.

31. Martinez AS, Saef J, Paszczuk A, et al. Implementation of a pharmacist-managed heart failure medication titration clinic. Am J Health Syst Pharm 2013;70(12):1070–6.

32. Gattis WA, Hasselblad V, Whellan DJ, et al. Reduction in heart failure events by the addition of a clinical pharmacist to the heart failure management team: results of the Pharmacist in Heart Failure Assessment Recommendation and Monitoring (PHARM) Study. Arch Intern Med 1999;159(16): 1939–45.

33. Slyer JT, Ferrara LR. The effectiveness of group visits for patients with heart failure on knowledge, quality of life, self-care, and readmissions: a systematic review protocol. JBI Libr Syst Rev 2012;10(58): 4647–58.

34. Kelkar AA, Spertus J, Pang P, et al. Utility of patient-reported outcome instruments in heart failure. JACC Heart Fail 2016;4(3):165–75.

35. Raphael C, Briscoe C, Davies J, et al. Limitations of the New York Heart Association functional classification system and self-reported walking distances in chronic heart failure. Heart (British Cardiac Society) 2007;93(4):476–82.

36. Calkins DR, Rubenstein LV, Cleary PD, et al. Failure of physicians to recognize functional disability in ambulatory patients. Ann Intern Med 1991;114(6): 451–4.

37. Weldring T, Smith SMS. Patient-reported outcomes (PROs) and patient-reported outcome measures (PROMs). Health Serv insights 2013;6:61–8.

38. Garin O, Herdman M, Vilagut G, et al. Assessing health-related quality of life in patients with heart failure: a systematic, standardized comparison of available measures. Heart Fail Rev 2014;19(3):359–67.

39. Bilbao A, Escobar A, García-Perez L, et al. The Minnesota Living with Heart Failure Questionnaire: comparison of different factor structures. Health Qual Life Outcomes 2016;14:23.

40. Napier R, McNulty SE, Eton DT, et al. Comparing measures to assess health-related quality of life in heart failure with preserved ejection fraction. JACC Heart Fail 2018;6(7):552–60.

41. Gonzalez-Saenz de Tejada M, Bilbao A, Ansola L, et al. Responsiveness and minimal clinically important difference of the Minnesota Living with Heart Failure Questionnaire. Health Qual Life Outcomes 2019;17(1):36.

42. Ni H, Toy W, Burgess D, et al. Comparative responsiveness of Short-Form 12 and Minnesota Living with Heart Failure Questionnaire in patients with heart failure. J Card Fail 2000;6(2):83–91.

43. Moser DK, Yamokoski L, Sun JL, et al. Improvement in health-related quality of life after hospitalization predicts event-free survival in patients with advanced heart failure. J Card Fail 2009;15(9): 763–9.

44. Green CP, Porter CB, Bresnahan DR, et al. Development and evaluation of the Kansas City

Cardiomyopathy Questionnaire: a new health status measure for heart failure. J Am Coll Cardiol 2000; 35(5):1245–55.

45. Heidenreich PA, Spertus JA, Jones PG, et al. Health status identifies heart failure outpatients at risk for hospitalization or death. J Am Coll Cardiol 2006; 47(4):752–6.

46. Spertus J, Peterson E, Conard MW, et al. Monitoring clinical changes in patients with heart failure: a comparison of methods. Am Heart J 2005;150(4): 707–15.

47. Kosiborod M, Soto GE, Jones PG, et al. Identifying heart failure patients at high risk for near-term cardiovascular events with serial health status assessments. Circulation 2007;115(15):1975–81.

48. Spertus JA, Jones PG. Development and validation of a short version of the Kansas City Cardiomyopathy Questionnaire. Circ Cardiovasc Qual Outcomes 2015;8(5):469–76.

49. Wohlfahrt PZS, Slager S, Allen LA, et al. Provider perspectives on the feasibility and utility of routine patient-reported outcomes assessment in heart failure: a qualitative analysis. J Am Heart Assoc 2020; 9(2):e013047.

50. Dickinson MG, Allen LA, Albert NA, et al. Remote monitoring of patients with heart failure: a White Paper From the Heart Failure Society of America Scientific Statements Committee. J Card Fail 2018;24(10): 682–94.

51. Inglis SC, Clark RA, Dierckx R, et al. Structured telephone support or non-invasive telemonitoring for patients with heart failure. Cochrane Database Syst Rev 2015;(10):CD007228.

52. Chaudhry SI, Mattera JA, Curtis JP, et al. Telemonitoring in patients with heart failure. N Engl J Med 2010;363(24):2301–9.

53. Koehler F, Winkler S, Schieber M, et al. Impact of remote telemedical management on mortality and hospitalizations in ambulatory patients with chronic heart failure: the telemedical interventional monitoring in heart failure study. Circulation 2011; 123(17):1873–80.

54. Ong MK, Romano PS, Edgington S, et al. Effectiveness of remote patient monitoring after discharge of hospitalized patients with heart failure: the Better Effectiveness After Transition–Heart Failure (BEAT-HF) Randomized Clinical Trial. JAMA Intern Med 2016;176(3):310–8.

55. Takahashi PY, Pecina JL, Upatising B, et al. A randomized controlled trial of telemonitoring in older adults with multiple health issues to prevent hospitalizations and emergency department visits. Arch Intern Med 2012;172(10):773–9.

56. Boyne JJ, Vrijhoef HJ, Crijns HJ, et al. Tailored telemonitoring in patients with heart failure: results of a multicentre randomized controlled trial. Eur J Heart Fail 2012;14(7):791–801.

57. Rahimi K, Velardo C, Triantafyllidis A, et al. A user-centred home monitoring and self-management system for patients with heart failure: a multicentre cohort study. Eur Heart J Qual Care Clin Outcomes 2015;1(2):66–71.

58. Hawkins NM, Virani SA, Sperrin M, et al. Predicting heart failure decompensation using cardiac implantable electronic devices: a review of practices and challenges. Eur J Heart Fail 2016;18(8):977–86.

59. Yu C-M, Wang L, Chau E, et al. Intrathoracic impedance monitoring in patients with heart failure. correlation with fluid status and feasibility of early warning preceding hospitalization. Circ J 2005;112(6):841–8.

60. Conraads VM, Tavazzi L, Santini M, et al. Sensitivity and positive predictive value of implantable intrathoracic impedance monitoring as a predictor of heart failure hospitalizations: the SENSE-HF trial. Eur Heart J 2011;32(18):2266–73.

61. Heist EK, Herre JM, Binkley PF, et al. Analysis of different device-based intrathoracic impedance vectors for detection of heart failure events (from the Detect Fluid Early from Intrathoracic Impedance Monitoring study). Am J Cardiol 2014;114(8): 1249–56.

62. Boehmer JP, Hariharan R, Devecchi FG, et al. A multisensor algorithm predicts heart failure events in patients with implanted devices. Results from the MultiSENSE Study. JACC Heart Fail 2017;5(3): 216–25.

63. Abraham WT, Adamson PB, Bourge RC, et al. Wireless pulmonary artery haemodynamic monitoring in chronic heart failure: a randomised controlled trial. Lancet 2011;377(9766):658–66.

64. Abraham WT, Stevenson LW, Bourge RC, et al. Sustained efficacy of pulmonary artery pressure to guide adjustment of chronic heart failure therapy: complete follow-up results from the CHAMPION randomised trial. Lancet 2016;387(10017): 453–61.

65. Pokharel Y, Khariton Y, Tang Y, et al. Association of serial Kansas City Cardiomyopathy Questionnaire assessments with death and hospitalization in patients with heart failure with preserved and reduced ejection fraction: a secondary analysis of 2 randomized clinical trials. JAMA Cardiol 2017;2(12): 1315–21.

Transitioning Patients with Heart Failure to Outpatient Care

R. Kannan Mutharasan, MD, FACC

KEYWORDS

- Heart failure • Transitional care • Readmissions • Process of care • Quality of care

KEY POINTS

- The transition from hospital to home is a vulnerable time for patients with heart failure. Specific processes of care should be built to ensure successful transition.
- Critical dimensions of success during the transitional care period include orienting properly to the patient's situation, ensuring discharge readiness, setting up feedback loops and monitoring parameters during transitional care, and successfully converting the patient to a chronic, outpatient mode of care.
- By examining the components of a prototypical feedback loop, local teams can determine what role any new technologies such as mobile health should play in future processes to support transitional care.
- Local teams should construct a process that makes sense given local resources and culture. It is impossible to do everything: the key is to build something that draws on strengths.

INTRODUCTION

The transition from hospitalization to outpatient care is a vulnerable time for patients with heart failure. The statistics are sobering: 30-day mortality is approximately 9%,[1] and 30-day readmissions rates remain high at 15% to 20%.[2,3] Home-time, a newer patient-centric metric, tells the same story. Patients recently hospitalized with heart failure and an ejection fraction less than or equal to 40% can expect to spend only 22 out of their next 30 days at home.[1] Examining a longer period postdischarge yields even more sobering insights. Patients who survive the 30-day period have a 1-year unadjusted mortality exceeding 30% and a 5-year mortality of about 75%.[4]

However the metrics for success are defined, transition to home is a transition that often fails. Numerous transitional care strategies can be deployed including patient education, medication reconciliation, care coordination postdischarge, telehealth interventions, and postdischarge follow-up appointments. Several recent systematic reviews have surveyed the heart failure transitional care literature.[5–8] These reviews demonstrate that, depending on the set of interventions selected, process improvements can have modest effects on meaningful transitional care outcomes. It is not yet clear what intervention or set of interventions are most impactful; in fact, this question is a focus of an upcoming trial.[9]

The literature is a guide for creating impactful transitional care programs on the ground. As a practical matter, interventions have to be adapted to the local environment to take effect.[10,11] The focus of this article is to provide a framework within which local care teams can develop programs to help patients successfully navigate the challenging transition from hospital to home.

Funding: The author received no funding.
Northwestern University Feinberg School of Medicine, 676 North Saint Clair Street, Arkes Pavilion, Suite 6-071, Chicago, IL 60611, USA
E-mail address: kannanm@northwestern.edu

We conceptualize the transition to home as having 4 steps (**Fig. 1**): (1) orienting properly to the patient, (2) ensuring discharge readiness, (3) developing feedback loops for course correction during transitional care, and (4) successfully transitioning the patient to a chronic, outpatient mode of therapy. Here we highlight existing evidence and process improvements that can support each stage.

STEP 1: TAKE A BROAD VIEW OF THE PATIENT, RECOGNIZING MEDICAL COMORBIDITIES AND SOCIOECONOMIC FACTORS. TAKE A DEEP VIEW OF HEART FAILURE, INVESTIGATING ROOT CAUSES

Patients admitted to the hospital with acute decompensated heart failure have many comorbidities.[12,13] For example, in a recently updated cohort of hospitalized patients with heart failure, the incidence of diabetes is nearly 40%, hypertension is 78%, atrial fibrillation is 41%, and coronary artery disease is 52%.[14] Reflecting this substantial burden of comorbid disease, only 35% of readmissions after hospitalization for heart failure are for recurrent heart failure.[15] These data underscore the need to link patients' primary care physicians into the plan of care. Indeed, the simple act of sending a discharge summary to the primary care physician is associated with lower readmission risk.[16]

Poverty can compound these comorbidities. Patients of low socioeconomic status face multiple barriers to accessing health care, and this is reflected in higher readmission rates after heart failure hospitalization for patients of low socioeconomic status[17] and is associated with higher mortality.[18] These medical and socioeconomic comorbidities indicate that heart failure is only one aspect of the typical heart failure patient's profile. Success means treating patients holistically, addressing multiple aspects of their care simultaneously.

At the same time, it is important to bear in mind that heart failure is a syndrome, not a diagnosis.

Multiple root causes can drive the syndrome, including valvular heart disease, ischemic heart disease, and hypertension. Addressing these more specific problems can help. From a process standpoint, efforts to identify and address the root cause can be regarded as a way to take variability out of the system, which will improve system reliability downstream. Thus, even as we take a holistic view of the patient, we must simultaneously try to define the underpinnings of the heart failure syndrome with as much specificity as possible.

STEP 2: ENSURE THE PATIENT IS READY FOR DISCHARGE FROM THE HEART FAILURE HOSPITALIZATION
Discharge Readiness

Discharge readiness remains an elusive concept. Galvin and colleagues[19] have framed this as ensuring that the patient is (1) physically stable, (2) has adequate support, (3) feels psychologically ready, and (4) has adequate information and knowledge to manage the disease. Note that only one of these components—physical stability—pertains to the illness itself. In the context of a patient with heart failure, this can be taken to mean the patient has adequate physical function to accomplish activities of daily living, has been appropriately decongested, and any root causes of the heart failure syndrome have been corrected or stabilized.

Decongestion

Decongestion, rather than clinical improvement, should be the goal of the heart failure hospitalization than symptom improvement. Several lines of evidence point to this. First, improved decongestion is associated with lower readmission rates.[20,21] For example, a subanalysis of the Acute Study of Clinical Effectiveness of Nesiritide in Decompensated Heart Failure (ASCEND-HF) trial observed that the absence of orthopnea, jugular venous distension, or rales was associated with a lower risk of readmission.[22] Second, decreased

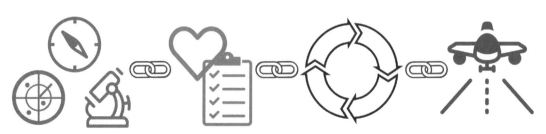

Orient to the Patient   Ensure Discharge Readiness   Set Up Feedback Loops   Stick the Landing

Fig. 1. Successful transition of patients to outpatient care.

levels of brain natriuretic peptide at discharge are associated with improved outcomes after heart failure hospitalization.[23] Third, hemoconcentration during the hospitalization is associated with better outcomes.[24]

Whether complete euvolemia or symptomatic improvement is the goal depends on many factors including the brittleness of the patient's volume status, the trajectory of diuresis, the ability of the patient to adhere to the treatment plan, and the availability of timely follow-up. For example, Bhatt and colleagues[25] found in a single-center study that cardiologists were more apt to discharge a patient early, potentially because of an increased ability to deliver more timely follow-up as compared with hospitalists. Bedside assessment of decongestion is likely to evolve, including techniques such as point-of-care ultrasound to assess inferior vena cava diameter.[26]

Medications

Discharge medications represent another pillar of readiness to discharge. The hospitalization offers opportunity to initiate and titrate a regimen of home medications. However, it seems to be just as common that medical therapy for heart failure is *de-escalated* during the hospitalization as it is for medical therapy to be *escalated*.[27] In heart failure with reduced ejection fraction (HFrEF), medication initiation in hospital is associated with better outcomes, whereas medication deescalation is associated with worse mortality.[28] Before discharge, observing the tolerability of the home regimen for 24 hours before discharge may be helpful,[29] although data are sparse regarding the clinical impact of this strategy.[25,30] It is emerging from contemporary registry data that medication tolerance is a major issue thwarting escalation of medication doses to target.[27] This underscores the necessity of medication counseling so that patients know what to expect with their new medication regimen.

In addition to focusing on guideline-directed medical therapy—a strategy that is disease modifying in the long run—it is also critical at hospital discharge to construct a diuretic management plan with the patient, because recurrent congestion will bring the patient back to the hospital. The home environment is very different from the hospital; thus, even the most carefully selected home-going dose of diuretic may be either too much or too little.

Selecting the correct medication profile for the patient is necessary but insufficient. Clinical teams must also pay careful attention to the mechanics of medication administration. Medication regimens for patients with heart failure are often bewilderingly complex, needing multiple medications dosed carefully throughout the day. Managing this poses significant logistical challenges for patients. It has been said that telecommunications has a "last mile" problem. In medicine, we have a "last yard" problem: getting medications from the pill bottle into the gastrointestinal tract. This chain of correct prescribing is fraught with error, involving prescriber error (prescriber prescribes the wrong medications), system error (the health care system because of insurance or other barriers cannot deliver the medications), and patient error (the patient does not know how to or chooses not to adhere to the prescribed regimen). Indeed, discrepancies in discharge medications are found in *half* of all patients discharged after hospitalization, with about half of this error on the system side and half on the patient side.[31]

Cardiovascular team–based interventions, including pharmacists[32] or nurses,[33] can assist with both the titration aspects and logistical aspects of medication management. The central idea is to assist patients with knowing their correct medications and assisting them by setting up pillboxes or blister packs of their scheduled medications. Patients do not just want to know what to take: they also want to know how the medications prescribed will help them. Thus, coupling medication interventions with patient education, using strategies such as the teach-back method,[34] is important.

Medical Comorbidities

Patients with heart failure also generally have multiple comorbid diseases, any of which could precipitate rehospitalization. Patients with HFpEF have more comorbidity-related readmissions than patients with HFrEF.[35] Coordinating care with primary care physicians and other subspecialists is essential. Although sometimes a simple phone call often is enough, more complex patients require more complex care coordination. There is an increasing interest toward patient-centered care and care redesign. Models such as the patient-centered specialty practice[36] or the dyspnea clinic[37] may help bring resources around a patient in a "pit stop" model, rather than have the patient go to different facilities to collect the care they need.

Social Factors

Beyond the medical illnesses described earlier, assessment of readiness for discharge should also include a social evaluation, coupled with attempts to address any barriers that are found.

Patients of all income strata, but particularly poor patients, face numerous barriers to attaining optimal health. Health literacy factors are strong among these barriers, often stopping patients from adhering to complex medication regimens,[38] particularly diuretics with often-changing doses.[39] Lack of social support has also been associated with worse outcomes after heart failure hospitalization.[40] Lack of insurance also often stops patients from getting to appointments or getting their critical medications.

These barriers can be challenging for health care providers to elicit. Patients may feel shame that they do not understand the medical plan or that they do not have the means to afford their medications.[40] An empathetic, nonjudgmental approach is critical. It is important to avoid the easy explanation of medication or dietary nonadherence and seek deeper root causes to address. Does the patient live in a food desert, and are there social programs that can work to help deliver healthier food? Can a pill box be supplied, and can the patient be coached in its use? Patients wish to get well; often there are simple barriers that thwart their efforts. There are few studies studying the impact of a social work intervention in isolation. However, the general medicine literature suggests that social workers are important members of transitional care teams to help reduce readmissions.[41]

What process improvements can be used to structure the implementation of discharge readiness?

Communication Tools: Handoffs, Checklists, and Audit and Feedback

Discharge summaries are the major way outpatient clinicians learn about what happened during their patients' hospitalizations. Thus, it is vital that this document be completed in a timely manner and forwarded to treating physicians before discharge. A challenge is that crucial information such as medication lists, problem lists, and treatments provided can be hard to find in the discharge summary in the era of electronic health record–facilitated note bloat. Furthermore, the outpatient physician will want to know not just what changes were made to medications but the rationale behind them.[42] To address this challenge, Hollenberg and colleagues[43] advocate for a focused discharge handoff that delivers critical clinical information about the patient recently hospitalized with heart failure. Such succinct communications tools are forward facing and provide relevant information formatted for action—in contrast to discharge summaries that often read as retrospective narratives of an often winding hospital course.

Checklists may be helpful in promoting quality of care for hospitalized patients with heart failure. From OPTIMIZE-HF registry data,[44] the use of checklists is associated with improved hospitalized heart failure outcomes. However, trial evidence in this space is sparse.[45,46] Discharge checklists for patients with heart failure, such as the one provided through the American Heart Association (AHA) Target:HF program,[47] can help organize the complex set of interventions that need to be delivered to patients with heart failure.

Over a longer timescale—weeks to months—audit and feedback of medical records back to clinicians regarding gaps in care can have significant impact on clinician and institutional performance.[48] Such programs include the American Heart Association Heart Failure Get With the Guidelines (AHA GWTG-HF). Through systematic chart review process and outcome metrics are measured and compiled. Doing so makes gaps in care visible both to individual practitioners as well as hospital systems. This in turn allows both individual clinicians and health systems to learn and build better frameworks for care delivery. The results of such a mechanism are impressive. Over the span of more than a decade now, there have been significant, sustained improvements on a variety of measures. At an individual hospital or hospital system level, engaging in programs such as AHA GWTG-HF helps provide structure to process improvement initiatives. Another benefit is that such programs can help provide external impetus to catalyze internal change management efforts.

STEP 3: SET UP FEEDBACK LOOPS FOR COURSE CORRECTION DURING TRANSITIONAL CARE
Transitional Care: a Vulnerable Period

The time from leaving the hospital and arriving in clinic at the next appointment is an incredibly vulnerable period for patients transitioning to outpatient care. During this time patients are in the blind spot of the medical system. When patients are home after the hospital stay, they often do not know whom to call with questions, find that there are issues with their medications, or do not fully understand the plan of care, which can be overwhelming. Furthermore, the home environment is often very different than the hospital environment. For example, diuretics carefully titrated in the hospital against sodium and fluid restrictions may be inadequate in the face of the home diet. Reflecting this, the most common day for rehospitalization after a heart failure admission is day 3 postdischarge.[15] The time from leaving the hospital to arriving to the first clinic visit is not a time for "set it and forget it." It is a time for feedback loops.

Feedback Loops

Feedback loops are mechanisms by which a system can be controlled. From a process control standpoint, after hospital discharge a major goal for heart failure care is to ensure that the patient's volume status remains stable or improves. Doing this requires at least 6 elements (**Fig. 2**).[49] Let us take the simple example of instructing a patient to monitor weight daily soon after hospital discharge—the limited evidence for efficacy of this strategy notwithstanding.[50] First is the parameter to be controlled. In this example, this is the morning weight. There must be a detector to detect the perturbation—in this case a scale. There must be means of communication back to the controlling center—in this case a telephone call or an electronic message. There must be a coordinating center to execute a computational step, for example, a nurse consulting with a physician to determine a better dose of diuretic or the patient consulting a variable diuretic dosing scheme. There must then be outbound communication of what action should be taken to address the perturbation, for example, instructions to double the dose of loop diuretic. Finally, there must be an effector mechanism to control the observed deviation from the expected weight: the patient must take the pill.

Examination of this control loop leads to several critical insights. First, without any component of the loop it is not possible to exert feedback control in the desired behavior. Each step in this chain is necessary. Second, the control loop is only as reliable as its weakest link. Third, the components of the feedback loop are modular. For example, a nurse could communicate back to a patient with instructions either by telephone or secure electronic message. This modularity means the feedback system can—and should—evolve as technology enables. Finally, time is a variable at play. Systems that respond more quickly are in general more effective and have reduced risk of reacting to old information. With this general construct in mind, we can now turn to examining potential elements of a course-correcting feedback loop during the time from hospital discharge to first clinic appointment.

Selected Feedback Mechanisms

Follow-up phone call

A postdischarge telephone call 48 to 72 hours after discharge helps care teams create a connection with patients, facilitating the feedback loop. A call in this timeframe serves several purposes. Defects in care, such as missing prescriptions or forgotten follow-up appointments can be addressed.[51] Learnings in the hospital can be reinforced and built on, interrupting the forgetting curve. Although phone call interventions have not been rigorously tested independently, they are common components of transitional care interventions for heart failure, which overall likely have moderate benefit.[8] Thus they continue to be a major point of emphasis in guidelines for transitional care of patients with heart failure.[43]

Symptom response

One potential "detector" of incipient congestion is patient self-awareness of symptoms. Different patients seem to exhibit different sensitivities to internal signals of feeling unwell.[52] The onset of congestion can be subtle; in fact data demonstrate that this is a lagging indicator as compared with increase in ventricular filling pressures.[53] Nonetheless it does seem that symptoms of congestion begin approximately a week before the need for heart failure hospitalization. Patients should be encouraged to bring symptoms to medical attention when they begin

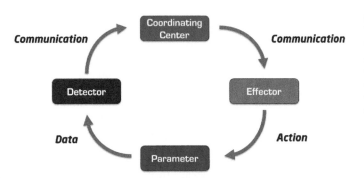

Fig. 2. A prototypical feedback loop. This comprises (1) a parameter to be controlled, (2) a detector, (3) communication back to a coordinating center, (4) a coordinating center, (5) communication out to an effector, and (6) an effector to get the controlled parameter back to baseline.

to feel unwell. At this stage it is possible that outpatient management can prevent recurrent hospitalization. Sensing symptoms and seeking care is a pattern of self-care behavior associated with improved heart failure outcomes.[52] One commonly used visual communication tool is the heart failure zone guide, dividing symptoms into green, yellow, and red zones.[34] This simple visual communication allows patients to quickly link signs and symptoms to appropriate clinical actions. In our experience, it is vitally important to emphasize to patients that they are not bothering their health care providers and that they will not be judged for becoming symptomatic. Patients can often feel a deep sense of shame, particularly if they feel that their behaviors contributed to symptoms. Addressing this up front can help lines of communication open and keep the feedback loop intact.

Daily weights

Daily weights are a very insensitive tool for detecting heart failure hospitalization, with some estimates as low as 9% sensitivity.[54] More than 50% of patients gain less than 1 kg before heart failure hospitalization. Nonetheless, in the absence of more advanced monitoring strategies, this simple tool may help avert some episodes of congestion. Although specific cut-points vary, patients should be instructed to call or to increase loop diuretic dose per rescue protocol if they encounter a 1.5 kg weight gain over 24 hours.

Devices for invasive cardiac monitoring

Because that weight gain is a lagging rather than a leading indicator of cardiac congestion, systems that allow for direct measurement of cardiac filling pressures may help avert heart failure hospitalizations. Multiple such devices have been studied, including implantable devices measuring the pressure in cardiac chambers and the use of algorithms on implantable cardioverter defibrillators to detect volume overload.[55] Among devices, the best studied is the CardioMEMS device (Abbott, Inc., Atlanta, GA, USA). This device is implanted into the left pulmonary artery and transmits pulmonary artery pressure readings. There is now accumulated trial[56] and real-world[57] evidence supporting the efficacy of pulmonary artery pressure–guided heart failure management. The benefit of this system seems to be largely driven by ability to better adjust medications, particularly loop diuretics.[58] In one study better outcomes were associated with more frequent daily transmissions,[59] underscoring the concept that a complete feedback loop is necessary to affect change.

STEP 4: "STICK THE LANDING"—CONVERT THE PATIENT TO A CHRONIC MODE OF THERAPY

The ultimate goal of transitional care is for a patient to enter an outpatient mode of therapy. Thirty days is a commonly accepted window, although there is no strict definition of the duration. An important first step in this transition—and often a rate-limiting step—is arriving to the posthospitalization clinic visit. American College of Cardiology/AHA guidelines recommend a 7-day post-hospital follow-up visit.[29] Yet the AHA-GWTG registry demonstrate that scheduled 7-day follow-up rates are low and arrivals to the 7-day appointment are dismal at 30%.[60]

We believe this is a process of care problem that can yield to insights offered by queuing theory, the mathematical study of waiting times.[61] One major insight queuing theory offers is that if you have a variable process (number of heart failure discharges from the hospital each day) feeding into a fixed capacity (number of discharge clinic slots per day), you need to have a *capacity buffer* to accommodate the variability in demand. Simply matching average supply of clinic slots to average demand for clinic slots is not enough because wait times will spiral out of control (**Fig. 3**). For example, queuing theory predicts that, under typical assumptions, a hospital clinic that is usedtilized to 99% capacity will only be able to accommodate 32% of patients within 7 days. If, however, the number of clinic slots is moderately expanded, then a significant number of patients can get into clinic within a 7-day window. For example, if utilization changes to 90% of capacity, 99% of patients will be accommodated within 7 days.[62] This is a significant improvement in performance for a modest modification to process. Those interested in deploying the queuing model to redesign clinic capacity can do so at a free online calculator located at http://hfresearch.org.

The post-hospital follow-up appointment is a useful checkpoint that serves at least 3 major purposes. The first is ensuring clinical stability. Diuretic therapy or other medications may need to be adjusted. A second major purpose is to reinforce education. Spaced repetition is a critical strategy to consolidate learning and interrupt the forgetting curve.[63] Finally, during the post-discharge follow-up visit the clinician can ensure that the patient is linked to other outpatient resources needed to ensure success, including primary care visits, home health, and cardiac rehabilitation.

This article began by zooming out and noting that patients hospitalized with heart failure carry multiple

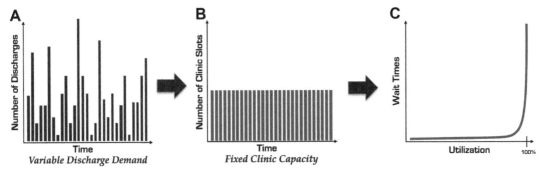

Fig. 3. The impact of variability on wait times. When a variable process such as discharges from a hospital (*A*) feed into a process with fixed capacity such as outpatient clinic (*B*), as utilization approaches 100%, wait times spiral out of control (*C*). A modest capacity buffer can significantly improve wait times.

comorbidities, any of which could result in a rehospitalization. Layered on top of this is the notion that hospitalization itself can engender frailty, a phenomenon termed posthospitalization syndrome.[64] This underscores the need for primary care and other specialty involvement to address comorbidities. Coordination of this care is complex. Yet it is critical that cardiovascular specialists engage in this coordination work—particularly because heart failure management needs frequent contact, which in turn engenders trust.

TOWARD THE FUTURE

The control loop framework helps visualize the impact new technology can have on transitional care. Understanding this can in turn help the transitional care team take advantage of new technologies to improve outcomes for patients and perhaps just as importantly empower teams to shun new technologies that do not help complete the feedback loop more quickly, reliably, safely, or more effectively.

To make this concrete, let us take the example of how new technologies as of this writing may affect volume management for recently discharged patients with heart failure. First, new wearable sensor technologies are being developed that may help *detect* decompensating patients with heart failure.[65,66] These data might be *communicated back* to a coordinating center using a patient's own mobile device passively, without any active intervention such as placing a telephone call. The *coordinating center* might use artificial intelligence to place the patient's device data into the global clinical context to ascertain whether and what kind of intervention is warranted. The *communication forward* to the patient might also proceed through the patient's own device. The *effector mechanism* might be a smart pill box that organizes medications well for the patient

and provides feedback to the provider about adherence to the therapy.

As technology advances, 3 major issues arise. The first is the issue of trust. Do we blindly trust the output of the algorithm? Or do we want human oversight, with a nurse or physician reviewing the recommendations before they are deployed? Does human oversight dilute the value of the algorithmic output?

The second is that the loop is only reliable as the weakest link. It is not sufficient to invest in improved detection technology without concomitant attention to communications tools and processes to manage the workflow and data. The whole feedback loop should be thought about holistically.

The third issue is that advances in technology will enable velocity, and this has the most disruptive potential. A benefit is that information and corrections can be delivered in small pieces during brief touchpoints. For example, one could envision heart failure education delivered on a mobile health platform in small daily "microlearnings."[63] A downside is that this potential velocity has no meaningful upper limit: computers can work tirelessly, processing and passing information on millisecond timescales. Without workflow enhancements to carefully curate the work requiring human intervention, this could become exhausting to providers.

CONCLUSION: WHAT ARE MY NEXT STEPS?

Here we offer a simple framework to guide development of a transitional care plan for patients with heart failure:

- Step 1: take a broad view of the patient, recognizing medical comorbidities and socioeconomic factors. Take a deep view of heart failure, investigating root causes.

- Step 2: ensure the patient is ready for discharge from the heart failure hospitalization.
- Step 3: set up feedback loops for course correction during transitional care.
- Step 4: "stick the landing"—convert the patient to a chronic mode of therapy.

Individual components of this are deceptively simple. The challenge is in creating a local team to design a pathway, collect the data, affect local change, measure the impact, and recalibrate.

For implementation, we offer 4 corresponding considerations:

1. Empower a local team and appoint a transitional care champion. Small dedicated teams can often achieve the focus needed to create large changes in organizations.[67] For example, at our center, we have developed a multidisciplinary team called the Heart Failure Bridge and Transition (BAT) team. The BAT team—consisting of a physician, 2 nurse practitioners, a pharmacist, a social worker, and 2 nurse coordinators—is tasked with the comprehensive discharge care of patients with heart failure. Based on CMS metrics, our center has continued to provide excellent, high-value care to hospitalized patients with heart failure.[68]
2. Start somewhere. Starting with a known problem and delivering quick wins builds team capacity and morale and creates belief that larger process improvements can be effectively tackled.
3. Do not try to do everything. There are a variety of potentially useful interventions to help patients transition to an outpatient setting. Not all of these will fit the local practice environment. For example, rural centers may invest more heavily in telehealth interventions because of the distance patients need to travel. Suburban centers with ample parking and short drives may choose to emphasize in-person visits.
4. Have a framework that addresses all components of the feedback loop. The feedback loop (see **Fig. 2**) can be a useful tool to diagnose weak links in the process and help guide which aspects require more attention for improvement.

In summary, process improvement lenses can help design more effective transitional care interventions for patients with heart failure. This framework can also help heart failure teams understand the potential impact of technology on patient care.

DISCLOSURE

The author has nothing to disclose.

REFERENCES

1. Greene SJ, O'Brien EC, Mentz RJ, et al. Home-time after discharge among patients hospitalized with heart failure. J Am Coll Cardiol 2018;71(23): 2643–52.
2. Kwok CS, Seferovic PM, Van Spall HG, et al. Early unplanned readmissions after admission to hospital with heart failure. Am J Cardiol 2019;124(5): 736–45.
3. Fonarow GC, Konstam MA, Yancy CW. The hospital readmission reduction program is associated with fewer readmissions, more deaths: time to reconsider. J Am Coll Cardiol 2017;70(15):1931–4.
4. Pandey A, Patel KV, Liang L, et al. Association of hospital performance based on 30-day risk-standardized mortality rate with long-term survival after heart failure hospitalization: an analysis of the get with the guidelines-heart failure registry. JAMA Cardiol 2018;3(6):489–97.
5. Albert NM. A systematic review of transitional-care strategies to reduce rehospitalization in patients with heart failure. Heart Lung 2016;45(2):100–13.
6. Van Spall HGC, Rahman T, Mytton O, et al. Comparative effectiveness of transitional care services in patients discharged from the hospital with heart failure: a systematic review and network meta-analysis. Eur J Heart Fail 2017;19(11):1427–43.
7. Albert NM, Barnason S, Deswal A, et al. Transitions of care in heart failure: a scientific statement from the American Heart Association. Circ Heart Fail 2015;8(2):384–409.
8. Takeda A, Martin N, Taylor RS, et al. Disease management interventions for heart failure. Cochrane Database Syst Rev 2019;(1):CD002752.
9. DeVore AD, Granger BB, Fonarow GC, et al. Care optimization through patient and hospital engagement clinical trial for heart failure: rationale and design of CONNECT-HF. Am Heart J 2019;220: 41–50.
10. Rabin BA, McCreight M, Battaglia C, et al. Systematic, multimethod assessment of adaptations across four diverse health systems interventions. Front Public Health 2018;6:102.
11. Wiltsey Stirman S, Baumann AA, Miller CJ. The FRAME: an expanded framework for reporting adaptations and modifications to evidence-based interventions. Implement Sci 2019;14(1):58.
12. Adams KF, Fonarow GC, Emerman CL, et al. Characteristics and outcomes of patients hospitalized for heart failure in the United States: rationale, design, and preliminary observations from the first 100,000 cases in the Acute Decompensated Heart

Failure National Registry (ADHERE). Am Heart J 2005;149(2):209–16.

13. Greene SJ, Butler J, Albert NM, et al. Medical therapy for heart failure with reduced ejection fraction: the CHAMP-HF registry. J Am Coll Cardiol 2018; 72(4):351–66.

14. Ziaeian B, Hernandez AF, DeVore AD, et al. Long-term outcomes for heart failure patients with and without diabetes: from the get with the guidelines-heart failure registry. Am Heart J 2019;211:1–10.

15. Dharmarajan K, Hsieh AF, Lin Z, et al. Diagnoses and timing of 30-day readmissions after hospitalization for heart failure, acute myocardial infarction, or pneumonia. JAMA 2013;309(4):355–63.

16. Bradley EH, Curry L, Horwitz LI, et al. Hospital strategies associated with 30-day readmission rates for patients with heart failure. Circ Cardiovasc Qual Outcomes 2013;6(4):444–50.

17. Patil S, Shah M, Patel B, et al. Readmissions among patients admitted with acute decompensated heart failure based on income quartiles. Mayo Clin Proc 2019;94(10):1939–50.

18. Ahmad K, Chen EW, Nazir U, et al. Regional variation in the association of poverty and heart failure mortality in the 3135 counties of the united states. J Am Heart Assoc 2019;8(18):e012422.

19. Galvin EC, Wills T, Coffey A. Readiness for hospital discharge: a concept analysis. J Adv Nurs 2017; 73(11):2547–57.

20. Lala A, McNulty SE, Mentz RJ, et al. Relief and recurrence of congestion during and after hospitalization for acute heart failure: insights from Diuretic Optimization Strategy Evaluation in Acute Decompensated Heart Failure (DOSE-AHF) and Cardiorenal Rescue Study in Acute Decompensated Heart Failure (CARESS-HF). Circ Heart Fail 2015;8(4):741–8.

21. Ambrosy AP, Pang PS, Khan S, et al. Clinical course and predictive value of congestion during hospitalization in patients admitted for worsening signs and symptoms of heart failure with reduced ejection fraction: findings from the EVEREST trial. Eur Heart J 2013;34(11):835–43.

22. Fudim M, O'Connor CM, Dunning A, et al. Aetiology, timing and clinical predictors of early vs. late readmission following index hospitalization for acute heart failure: insights from ASCEND-HF. Eur J Heart Fail 2018;20(2):304–14.

23. Dhaliwal AS, Deswal A, Pritchett A, et al. Reduction in BNP levels with treatment of decompensated heart failure and future clinical events. J Card Fail 2009;15(4):293–9.

24. Greene SJ, Gheorghiade M, Vaduganathan M, et al. Haemoconcentration, renal function, and post-discharge outcomes among patients hospitalized for heart failure with reduced ejection fraction: insights from the EVEREST trial. Eur J Heart Fail 2013;15(12):1401–11.

25. Bhatt AB, Cheeran DD, Shemisa K, et al. Physician-specific practice patterns about discharge readiness and heart failure utilization outcomes. Circ Cardiovasc Qual Outcomes 2018;11(11):e004365.

26. Akhabue E, Pierce JB, Davidson LJ, et al. A prospective pilot study of pocket-carried ultrasound pre- and postdischarge inferior vena cava assessment for prediction of heart failure rehospitalization. J Card Fail 2018;24(9):614–7.

27. Greene SJ, Fonarow GC, DeVore AD, et al. Titration of medical therapy for heart failure with reduced ejection fraction. J Am Coll Cardiol 2019;73(19): 2365–83.

28. Tran RH, Aldemerdash A, Chang P, et al. Guideline-directed medical therapy and survival following hospitalization in patients with heart failure. Pharmacotherapy 2018;38(4):406–16.

29. Yancy CW, Jessup M, Bozkurt B, et al. 2013 ACCF/AHA guideline for the management of heart failure: a report of the American College of Cardiology Foundation/American Heart Association Task Force on Practice Guidelines. J Am Coll Cardiol 2013; 62(16):e147–239.

30. Laliberte B, Reed BN, Devabhakthuni S, et al. Observation of patients transitioned to an oral loop diuretic before discharge and risk of readmission for acute decompensated heart failure. J Card Fail 2017;23(10):746–52.

31. Milfred-LaForest SK, Gee JA, Pugacz AM, et al. Heart failure transitions of care: a pharmacist-led post-discharge pilot experience. Prog Cardiovasc Dis 2017;60(2):249–58.

32. Neu R, Leonard MA, Dehoorne ML, et al. Impact of pharmacist involvement in heart failure transition of care. Ann Pharmacother 2019. https://doi.org/10.1177/1060028019882685. 1060028019882685.

33. Driscoll A, Currey J, Tonkin A, et al. Nurse-led titration of angiotensin converting enzyme inhibitors, beta-adrenergic blocking agents, and angiotensin receptor blockers for people with heart failure with reduced ejection fraction. Cochrane Database Syst Rev 2015;(12):CD009889.

34. White M, Garbez R, Carroll M, et al. Is "teach-back" associated with knowledge retention and hospital readmission in hospitalized heart failure patients? J Cardiovasc Nurs 2013;28(2):137–46.

35. Ather S, Chan W, Bozkurt B, et al. Impact of noncardiac comorbidities on morbidity and mortality in a predominantly male population with heart failure and preserved versus reduced ejection fraction. J Am Coll Cardiol 2012;59(11):998–1005.

36. Ward L, Powell RE, Scharf ML, et al. Patient-centered specialty practice: defining the role of specialists in value-based health care. Chest 2017; 151(4):930–5.

37. Ryan JJ, Waxman AB. The Dyspnea clinic. Circulation 2018;137(19):1994–6.

38. McNaughton CD, Cawthon C, Kripalani S, et al. Health literacy and mortality: a cohort study of patients hospitalized for acute heart failure. J Am Heart Assoc 2015;4(5). https://doi.org/10.1161/JAHA.115.001799.

39. Retrum JH, Boggs J, Hersh A, et al. Patient-identified factors related to heart failure readmissions. Circ Cardiovasc Qual Outcomes 2013;6(2):171–7.

40. Kangovi S, Barg FK, Carter T, et al. Challenges faced by patients with low socioeconomic status during the post-hospital transition. J Gen Intern Med 2014;29(2):283–9.

41. Bellon JE, Bilderback A, Ahuja-Yende NS, et al. University of Pittsburgh medical center home transitions multidisciplinary care coordination reduces readmissions for older adults. J Am Geriatr Soc 2019;67(1):156–63.

42. Robelia PM, Kashiwagi DT, Jenkins SM, et al. Information transfer and the hospital discharge summary: national primary care provider perspectives of challenges and opportunities. J Am Board Fam Med 2017;30(6):758–65.

43. Hollenberg SM, Warner Stevenson L, Ahmad T, et al. 2019 ACC expert consensus decision pathway on risk assessment, management, and clinical trajectory of patients hospitalized with heart failure: a report of the american college of cardiology solution set oversight committee. J Am Coll Cardiol 2019;74(15):1966–2011.

44. Fonarow GC, Abraham WT, Albert NM, et al. Influence of a performance-improvement initiative on quality of care for patients hospitalized with heart failure: results of the Organized Program to Initiate Lifesaving Treatment in Hospitalized Patients with Heart Failure (OPTIMIZE-HF). Arch Intern Med 2007;167(14):1493–502.

45. Legallois D, Chaufourier L, Blanchart K, et al. Improving quality of care in patients with decompensated acute heart failure using a discharge checklist. Arch Cardiovasc Dis 2019;112(8-9):494–501.

46. Basoor A, Doshi NC, Cotant JF, et al. Decreased readmissions and improved quality of care with the use of an inexpensive checklist in heart failure. Congest Heart Fail 2013;19(4):200–6.

47. Target: HF Strategies and Clinical Tools | American Heart Association. Available at: https://www.heart.org/en/professional/quality-improvement/target-heart-failure/strategies-and-clinical-tools. Accessed January 16, 2020.

48. Ellrodt AG, Fonarow GC, Schwamm LH, et al. Synthesizing lessons learned from get with the guidelines: the value of disease-based registries in improving quality and outcomes. Circulation 2013;128(22):2447–60.

49. Boron WF. Medical physiology. 3rd edition. Philadelphia: Elsevier; 2017. p. 1312.

50. Jones CD, Holmes GM, DeWalt DA, et al. Self-reported recall and daily diary-recorded measures of weight monitoring adherence: associations with heart failure-related hospitalization. BMC Cardiovasc Disord 2014;14:12.

51. Johnson MB, Laderman M, Coleman EA. Enhancing the effectiveness of follow-up phone calls to improve transitions in care: three decision points. Jt Comm J Qual Patient Saf 2013;39(5):221–7.

52. Lee CS, Bidwell JT, Paturzo M, et al. Patterns of self-care and clinical events in a cohort of adults with heart failure: 1 year follow-up. Heart Lung 2018;47(1):40–6.

53. Zile MR, Bennett TD, St John Sutton M, et al. Transition from chronic compensated to acute decompensated heart failure: pathophysiological insights obtained from continuous monitoring of intracardiac pressures. Circulation 2008;118(14):1433–41.

54. Adamson PB. Pathophysiology of the transition from chronic compensated and acute decompensated heart failure: new insights from continuous monitoring devices. Curr Heart Fail Rep 2009;6(4):287–92.

55. Veenis JF, Brugts JJ. Remote monitoring of chronic heart failure patients: invasive versus non-invasive tools for optimising patient management. Neth Heart J 2020;28(1):3–13.

56. Abraham WT, Compton S, Haas G, et al. Intrathoracic impedance vs daily weight monitoring for predicting worsening heart failure events: results of the Fluid Accumulation Status Trial (FAST). Congest Heart Fail 2011;17(2):51–5.

57. Heywood JT, Jermyn R, Shavelle D, et al. Impact of practice-based management of pulmonary artery pressures in 2000 patients implanted with the CardioMEMS sensor. Circulation 2017;135(16):1509–17.

58. Costanzo MR, Stevenson LW, Adamson PB, et al. Interventions linked to decreased heart failure hospitalizations during ambulatory pulmonary artery pressure monitoring. JACC Heart Fail 2016;4(5):333–44.

59. Tran JS, Wolfson AM, O'Brien D, et al. A systems-based analysis of the CardioMEMS HF sensor for chronic heart failure management. Cardiol Res Pract 2019;2019:7979830.

60. DeVore AD, Cox M, Eapen ZJ, et al. Temporal trends and variation in early scheduled follow-up after a hospitalization for heart failure: findings from get with the guidelines-heart failure. Circ Heart Fail 2016;9(1). https://doi.org/10.1161/CIRCHEARTFAILURE.115.002344.

61. Anupindi R, Chopra S, Deshmukh SD, et al. Managing business process flows. 3rd edition. Boston: Pearson; 2012. p. 352.

62. Mutharasan RK, Ahmad FS, Gurvich I, et al. Buffer or suffer: redesigning heart failure postdischarge clinic

using queuing theory. Circ Cardiovasc Qual Outcomes 2018;11(7):e004351.

63. Shail MS. Using micro-learning on mobile applications to increase knowledge retention and work performance: a review of literature. Cureus 2019;11(8):e5307.

64. Krumholz HM. Post-hospital syndrome–an acquired, transient condition of generalized risk. N Engl J Med 2013;368(2):100–2.

65. Inan OT, Baran Pouyan M, Javaid AQ, et al. Novel wearable seismocardiography and machine learning algorithms can assess clinical status of heart failure patients. Circ Heart Fail 2018;11(1): e004313.

66. DeVore AD, Wosik J, Hernandez AF. The future of wearables in heart failure patients. JACC Heart Fail 2019;7(11):922–32.

67. Trimble C. The best way to improve health care delivery is with a small, dedicated team. Harv Bus Rev 2016. Available at: https://hbr.org/2016/03/the-best-way-to-improve-health-care-delivery-is-with-a-small-dedicated-team. Accessed January 15 2020.

68. Find and compare information about Hospitals | Hospital Compare. Available at: https://www.medicare.gov/hospitalcompare/search.html?. Accessed January 24, 2020.

Innovation in Ambulatory Care of Heart Failure in the Era of Coronavirus Disease 2019

Orly Leiva, MD[a,1], Ankeet S. Bhatt, MD, MBA[b,1], Muthiah Vaduganathan, MD, MPH[b,*]

KEYWORDS

- Ambulatory • Care optimization • COVID-19 • Guideline-directed medical therapy • Heart failure

KEY POINTS

- Major gaps exist in the implementation of guideline-directed medical therapy for heart failure (HF). Ambulatory care optimization should focus on rapid and successful implementation of effective therapies.
- HF is associated with high comorbid disease burden. Ambulatory management of comorbidities should be incorporated into HF disease management programs.
- Optimizing ambulatory HF care will require a multidisciplinary team to address therapeutic optimization, active comorbid disease management, and nutrition and structured exercise-based interventions.

INTRODUCTION

Heart failure (HF) is a chronic disease state that affects up to 6 million Americans; the prevalence is poised to rise in upcoming years given population aging and adverse trends in cardiometabolic comorbidities.[1] HF is a major contributor of morbidity and mortality in the United States, with 1 in 9 death certificates mentioning HF and more than 58,000 deaths attributed to HF annually.[1] The natural history of HF with reduced ejection fraction (HFrEF) has been significantly disrupted with the sequential development and demonstration of benefit of 6 distinct classes of disease-modifying therapies: angiotensin-converting enzyme inhibitors (ACEi), angiotensin II receptor blockers (ARB), angiotensin receptor-neprilysin inhibitors (ARNI), β-blockers, mineralocorticoid receptor antagonists (MRA), and most recently, the

sodium glucose cotransporter-2 inhibitors (SGLT2i). However, despite these recent advances, fewer than 1% of patients with HF are simultaneously treated with target doses of multiple evidence-based classes (ACEi/ARB/ARNI, β-blockers, and MRA).[2–4] In addition, as there are currently no approved therapies for patients with HF with preserved ejection fraction, its management has relied on the rigorous targeting of key comorbidities and effective hemodynamic and volume-control strategies.

Although focus on optimization around the time of hospitalization represents an important target of care efforts, a large segment of the HF population lives in community settings, at times with limited care access. Most patient-physician interactions occur in ambulatory clinics, including those that span primary care, cardiology, and advanced HF. As such, optimizing care pathways in the

[a] Department of Medicine, Brigham and Women's Hospital, Boston, MA, USA; [b] Division of Cardiovascular Medicine, Brigham and Women's Hospital, Boston, MA, USA
[1] Co-first authors.
* Corresponding author. 75 Francis Street, Boston, MA 02215.
E-mail address: mvaduganathan@bwh.harvard.edu
Twitter: @LeivaOrly (O.L.); @ankeetbhatt (A.S.B.); @mvaduganathan (M.V.)

Heart Failure Clin 16 (2020) 433–440
https://doi.org/10.1016/j.hfc.2020.06.004

ambulatory setting is a particularly promising area of care innovation. In addition, the emergence of the Coronavirus Disease 2019 (COVID-19) pandemic has threatened traditional care approaches, limiting health care access and interactions. The introduction of new technologies and expansion in insurance coverage of telehealth options, combined with team-based multidisciplinary efforts, have the potential to provide a lasting impact on care delivery in ambulatory practice.

GAPS IN PROVISION OF EVIDENCE-BASED THERAPIES

Data from the Changing the Management of Patients with Heart Failure (CHAMP-HF), Contemporary Drug Treatment of Chronic HF (CHECK-HF), and Quality of Adherence to guideline recommendations for life-saving treatment in HF survey (QUALIFY) registries suggest there are important gaps in the use and dosing of key elements of guideline-directed medical therapy (GDMT) in clinical practice.[5–9] Despite a robust evidence base and guideline documents supporting full implementation of GDMT at target doses, the administration and uptitration of these therapies in patients with HFrEF are suboptimal[10] (**Table 1**).

IMPLEMENTING GUIDELINE-DIRECTED MEDICAL THERAPY

Given the multifaceted interactions between patients with HF and the health care system, team-based care approaches to GDMT optimization may be particularly valuable.[11] One strategy to improve delivery of GDMT is using non-physician medical staff under the guidance of HF specialists to engage in more active and frequent therapeutic changes. For instance, clinical pharmacists are experienced members of inpatient and outpatient interdisciplinary care teams and may serve as an important resource to aid in earlier initiation and uptitration. A model of pharmacist involvement in HF consult services in the inpatient setting has led to increased use of GDMT.[12] In the outpatient setting, one small pilot study used pharmacists to help manage dose titrations of GDMT. Despite small sample size, this intervention led to target dose β-blocker titration in 78% of patients and a significant reduction in all-cause hospital admissions.[13] Other studies have also shown reduction in hospital readmissions for HF when pharmacists are used to assist GDMT implementation in the outpatient setting.[14] Similarly, nursing-directed clinics have also been shown to increase adherence and optimize titration of GDMT.[15,16] Organizing these non-physician providers in GDMT-specific clinics (**Fig. 1**) represents a strategy to de-link usual care (which may focus on acute care needs and decongestion) and therapeutic optimization.[17,18] Randomized clinical trials examining an early intensive GDMT uptitration strategy as compared with usual care are under way (NCT03412201).

High-Quality Transitions in Care

Quality improvement programs have been previously implemented to attempt to improve GDMT uptake in patients admitted with HF. The American Heart Association's Get with the Guidelines Heart Failure (GWTG-HF) program is one such example.[19] Hospitals participating in the GWTG-HF program had higher use of GDMT (notably ACEi) and slightly improved readmission rates.[20,21] The GWTG-HF program expands on the progress of preceding initiatives including the Organized Program to Initiate Lifesaving Treatment in Hospitalized Patients with Heart Failure (OPTIMIZE-HF) program, which focused on implementing high-quality care at hospital discharge.[22] Process improvement initiatives embedded within

Table 1
Incomplete use and target dose achievement of guideline-directed medical therapy for heart failure with reduced ejection fraction in usual care settings globally

Registry	On/Adherent to Therapy, %			≥50% Target Dose,[a] %			≥100% Target Dose,[a] %		
	ACEi/ ARB/ARNI	Beta Blocker	MRA	ACEi/ ARB/ARNI	Beta Blocker	MRA	ACEi/ ARB/ARNI	Beta Blocker	MRA
CHAMP-HF	73.4	67	33.4	83.1	72.5	98.2	16.8	27.5	76.6
CHECK-HF	84	86	56	76	55	97.9	43.6	18.9	52
QUALIFY	62	79	86	74	60	76	22.7	14.8	70.8

Abbreviations: ACEi, angiotensin-converting enzyme inhibitor; ARB, angiotensin receptor blocker; ARNI, angiotensin receptor-neprilysin inhibitor; CHAMP-HF, changing the management of patients with heart failure; CHECK-HF, Contemporary Drug Treatment of Chronic HF; MRA, mineralocorticoid receptor antagonist; QUALIFY, quality of adherence to guideline recommendations for life-saving treatment in HF survey.
[a] Percentages reported as a proportion of patients on therapy.

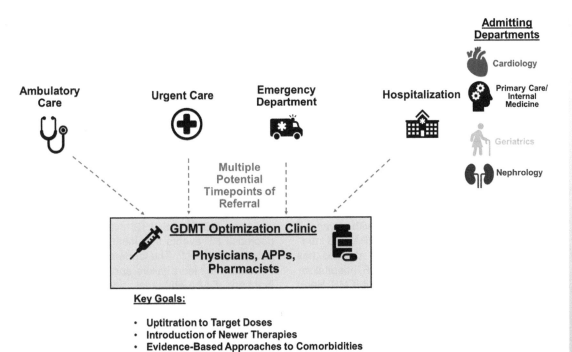

Fig. 1. Innovative care delivery pathway to optimize GDMT in HF. APP, advanced practice provider. (*From* Myhre PL, Januzzi JL Jr, Butler J, et al. De novo heart failure: where the journey begins. Eur J Heart Fail 2019, 21(10):1245–7; with permission.)

OPTIMIZE-HF were shown to be associated with reduced HF and cardiovascular readmission rates.[23] In parallel with these "real-world" clinical programs, traditional randomized trials have demonstrated that in-hospital initiation of evidence-based therapies is not only safe, but may lead to improved postdischarge use and therapeutic persistence.[24–26] However, patient-centered transitional care alone, such as evaluated in the Patient-Centered Care Transitions in HF (PACT-HF) service model, has not been associated with improved postdischarge outcomes.[27] In the PACT-HF trial the intervention group incorporated a hospital nurse navigator to facilitate a needs-based assessment and intervention reflecting self-reported quality of life, education, patient-centered discharge summary, multidisciplinary referrals, and family physician follow-up at the time of discharge. These findings highlight the importance of linked programs specifically designed to improve GDMT uptake during HF hospitalization, which seamlessly continue acceleration of therapy in the post-hospitalization period.

Telemedicine and Remote Health Management

Telemedicine represents an emerging strategy for optimizing GDMT and HF care at a more rapid pace, especially for patients who live in rural settings or those with limited access or high barriers to traditional clinical visits. These approaches may be particularly relevant in an era of COVID-19 and associated need for social distancing, further limiting contact with traditional ambulatory clinic settings. Indeed, the Centers for Medicare and Medicaid Services has expanded coverage to Medicare telehealth services in March 2020 in response to the escalating COVID-19 pandemic.

Although the results have been mixed in other clinical settings, studies suggest that telemedicine may facilitate improved patient interaction that may in turn promote GDMT initiation and uptitration at a scale difficult to obtain with traditional in-person visits.[28–30] A meta-analysis of 8323 patients across 25 randomized controlled trials suggested a reduction in all-cause mortality with telemonitoring (monitoring blood pressure, weight, electrocardiographic strips) compared with usual care among patients with HF.[31] In the Telemedical Interventional Management in Heart Failure II (TIM-HF2) trial conducted in Germany, patients with HF were randomized to telemonitoring strategy or usual care.[29] The telemonitoring group was given an electrocardiogram device, blood pressure measuring device, electronic scale, oximeter, and a mobile phone to communicate remotely with the clinic. The telemedical data were transmitted daily and the patient was managed according to a set algorithm. Telemonitoring reduced cardiovascular mortality and hospitalization for HF after 12 months of follow-up.[29] Given improvement in technology and continuous assessment, using wearable technology offers a new and convenient method for managing HF in the outpatient setting and particularly alerting providers when hemodynamics may allow for more aggressive GDMT. For example, one study provided participants a smartphone and a smartwatch along with an application that tracked participant activity data and required them to input daily self-measured blood pressure and body weight. Although this study was limited in size, a significant increase in quality of life and performance status was reported.[32] In patients with advanced HF, monitoring of pulmonary artery (PA) and intracardiac pressures via implantable devices has already been shown to reduce HF hospitalizations.[33,34] For example, the CardioMEMS Heart Sensor Allows Monitoring of Pressure to Improve Outcomes in NYHA Class III Heart Failure Patients (CHAMPION) trial showed improved clinical outcomes with longitudinal assessment and access to real-time PA pressure measurements that may be due to improved GDMT in the monitored group.[33] Given interconnectivity and telecommunication advances in the modern era, telemedicine is poised to become increasingly important in the management of chronic diseases such as HF. For example, the upcoming HF Study to Evaluate Vital Signs and Overcome Low Use of GDMT by Remote Monitoring (HF-eVOLUTION) trial will be evaluating the effectiveness of vital signs monitoring via wrist watch on GDMT use and may shed light on this novel strategy (NCT04292275). Similar telehealth solutions should be developed and empirically evaluated to determine if implementation may help improve GDMT use.

COMORBIDITY MANAGEMENT IN HEART FAILURE

Patients with HF often have comorbid noncardiac conditions that contribute to morbidity, mortality, and impaired health-related quality of life. In one study, more than 80% of patients with HF had at least 1 noncardiovascular comorbid condition and 25% had more than 3.[35] Patients with HF and comorbid conditions have worse outcomes, including increased mortality and HF admissions.[35] Chronic obstructive lung disease (COPD) and anemia have independently been associated with increased HF admissions and poorer outcomes.[36] Patients with comorbid conditions also had more severe HF symptoms, including fatigue, dyspnea, pain, and anxiety, which may collectively contribute to worse quality of life.[37] Therefore, comprehensive ambulatory management of patients with HF should include active surveillance and management of comorbid conditions. In addition, added comorbidity burden increased polypharmacy and may adversely affect adherence. Evaluation and early treatment or prevention of comorbid conditions are crucial to prevent potential exacerbation of HF and provide comprehensive cardiopulmonary and systemic care.

The most commonly identified comorbidities in patients with HF are diabetes mellitus, COPD, chronic kidney disease, and anemia.[35,37–39] In patients with diabetes mellitus (both with and without HF), new therapeutic options have emerged, including SGLT2i. SGLT2i has been found to decrease HF events in patients with type 2 diabetes mellitus.[40–44] The landmark Dapagliflozin in Patients with Heart Failure and Reduced Ejection Fraction (DAPA-HF) trial additionally demonstrated that dapagliflozin may be helpful in the treatment of patients with established HFrEF.[45] Cardiologists will need to take a more active role in prescribing these therapies, which have traditionally been considered only for their glucose-lowering potential. COPD is comorbid with HF and has been associated with increased mortality and hospitalization.[46,47] In the context of multiple intersecting comorbidities, programs designed to aid patients in medication adherence (and avoidance of potentially harmful or unnecessary therapies) will become increasingly important, particularly as medication burden increases.[48]

Last, depression is an often-overlooked comorbidity in patients with HF. Depression is comorbid in approximately 22% of patients with HF and has been associated with poor health-related quality of life and is an independent risk factor for subsequent cardiovascular events.[49,50] Importantly, depression may adversely impact therapeutic and lifestyle adherence.[51] Therefore, early screening and mental health support may be an additional avenue to improve adherence in patients with HF with concomitant depression.

VACCINATION

Vaccination is an important part of global prevention, even more so in patients with chronic diseases such as HF. In particular, vaccination against pulmonary pathogens (influenza and pneumococcus) in HF has some promise in improving outcomes, although no large clinical trials have been reported yet.[52] There are many plausible mechanisms by which influenza infection may promote worsening HF, including proinflammatory acceleration of atherogenesis in addition to direct myocardial depressant effects of inflammatory cytokines.

Routine early influenza vaccination has been shown to be effective in patients with atherosclerotic vascular disease and recent acute coronary syndrome.[53] In addition, recent data suggest that early, well-matched consistent influenza vaccination in patients with HF may improve clinical outcomes and reduce rehospitalization rates.[54] Data from a large randomized clinical trial also showed an association between influenza vaccination and improved cardiovascular events.[55] Despite this, usual care evidence suggests major gaps in influenza vaccination rates in the United States, with increasing refusal rates.[56] In addition, centers performing well with respect to influenza vaccination in patients with HF also performed well with respect to other HF quality measures, suggesting that particular centers may have integrated structured approaches to influenza vaccination administration into traditional HF disease management programs. Despite common sense indication for influenza vaccination and clear biological plausibility for benefit in patients with established cardiopulmonary disease, a focal anti-vaccination contingent and strong personal feelings and fears with regard to influenza vaccination may, in part, explain disappointing vaccination rates among patients with cardiovascular disease. New implementation avenues, particular those that may involve direct, patient-facing behavioral economic nudges, are needed to better understand barriers for nonvaccination and strategies for improvement. These learnings from vaccination efforts for seasonal influenza may be effectively translated to overcome upcoming challenges in disseminating effective vaccines against COVID-19 (once developed and available).

LIFESTYLE INTERVENTIONS IN AMBULATORY PRACTICE

As with many chronic cardiometabolic diseases, lifestyle modification is critical as a central tenet of disease management. HF is no exception, and thus lifestyle modification interventions should be part of every outpatient HF program and clinic. Structured exercise programs are one such intervention that has been proposed in HF, particularly given the overlap among HF, metabolic syndrome, and obesity, all of which are potentially mitigated by exercise and accelerated basal metabolic rates.[57] The Heart Failure: A Controlled Trial Investigating Outcomes of Exercise Training (HF-ACTION) trial investigated the health effects of an exercise training program in patients with HFrEF.[58] This trial showed that an exercise training program in patients with HF is safe and may have modest reductions in all-cause and cardiovascular mortality and hospitalization.[58] Patients in the exercise

group also had improved 6-minute walk distance and cardiopulmonary exercise duration. Furthermore, this improvement in 6-minute walk distance and cardiopulmonary exercise duration was similar across baseline physical activity levels.[59] One small study showed that a multidisciplinary clinic with cardiac rehabilitation, dieticians, psychologists, and nurse educators reduced HF hospitalization.[60] In addition to exercise, diet is important for HF and health overall.[61] HF is a catabolic state and malnutrition and cachexia are poor prognostic factors in HF.[62] One small upcoming study will investigate the role of diet optimization via nutrition education on nutritional and quality-of-life outcomes in patients with HF (NCT03845309), although larger trials are needed to investigate disruptive nutritional programs that may benefit patients with HF.

SUMMARY

Advancement in therapeutic options in recent decades have afforded us several avenues and tools for care optimization, including pharmacologic therapies, novel technology-based monitoring, and nonpharmacological interventions, such as vaccination, nutrition, and structured exercise-based approaches. Delivering high-quality HF care in a fragmented health system is increasingly challenging and likely ineffective; integrated ambulatory clinics designed around multidisciplinary teams including physicians, advanced practice providers, clinical pharmacists, nurses, nutritionists, exercise physiologists, and social workers, among others, are needed to provide care that is effective and optimal. These approaches, coupled with telehealth solutions, may minimize multiple health care interactions and travel for patients at risk for COVID-19. Furthermore, greater study is needed with regard to how these teams may effectively partner and engage patients to be champions of their own health, empowering them to seek new interventions, technologies, and lifestyle changes. Overall, the ambulatory setting (extending well beyond the walls of a single clinic) offers a comprehensive environment for care optimization. Ambulatory innovations in HF care must focus not only on disease-modifying interventions, but also on comprehensive HF and comorbid care designed to relieve symptoms, improve functional status, and optimize nutrition and weight management.

DISCLOSURE

O. Leiva and A.S. Bhatt have no relevant disclosures. M. Vaduganathan is supported by the

KL2/Catalyst Medical Research Investigator Training award from Harvard Catalyst (NIH/NCATS Award UL 1TR002541); serves on advisory boards for Amgen, AstraZeneca, Baxter Healthcare, Bayer AG, Boehringer Ingelheim, Cytokinetics, and Relypsa; and participates on clinical endpoint committees for studies sponsored by Novartis and the National Institutes of Health.

REFERENCES

1. Mozaffarian D, Benjamin EJ, Go AS, et al. Heart disease and stroke statistics–2015 update: a report from the American Heart Association. Circulation 2015;131(4):e29–322.

2. Greene SJ, Fonarow GC, DeVore AD, et al. Titration of medical therapy for heart failure with reduced ejection fraction. J Am Coll Cardiol 2019;73(19): 2365–83.

3. Peri-Okonny PA, Mi X, Khariton Y, et al. Target doses of heart failure medical therapy and blood pressure: insights from the CHAMP-HF registry. JACC Heart Fail 2019;7(4):350–8.

4. Bress AP, King JB. Optimizing medical therapy in chronic worsening HFrEF: a long way to go. J Am Coll Cardiol 2019;73(8):945–7.

5. DeVore AD, Thomas L, Albert NM, et al. Change the management of patients with heart failure: rationale and design of the CHAMP-HF registry. Am Heart J 2017;189:177–83.

6. Greene SJ, Butler J, Albert NM, et al. Medical therapy for heart failure with reduced ejection fraction: the CHAMP-HF registry. J Am Coll Cardiol 2018; 72(4):351–66.

7. Brunner-La Rocca HP, Linssen GC, Smeele FJ, et al. Contemporary drug treatment of chronic heart failure with reduced ejection fraction: the CHECK-HF registry. JACC Heart Fail 2019;7(1):13–21.

8. Komajda M, Cowie MR, Tavazzi L, et al. Physicians' guideline adherence is associated with better prognosis in outpatients with heart failure with reduced ejection fraction: the QUALIFY international registry. Eur J Heart Fail 2017;19(11):1414–23.

9. Komajda M, Anker SD, Cowie MR, et al. Physicians' adherence to guideline-recommended medications in heart failure with reduced ejection fraction: data from the QUALIFY global survey. Eur J Heart Fail 2016;18(5):514–22.

10. Yancy CW, Januzzi JL Jr, Allen LA, et al. 2017 ACC expert consensus decision pathway for optimization of heart failure treatment: answers to 10 pivotal issues about heart failure with reduced ejection fraction: a report of the American College of Cardiology Task Force on Expert Consensus Decision Pathways. J Am Coll Cardiol 2018;71(2): 201–30.

11. Wagner EH. The role of patient care teams in chronic disease management. BMJ 2000;320(7234):569–72.

12. Blizzard S, Verbosky N, Stein B, et al. Evaluation of pharmacist impact within an interdisciplinary inpatient heart failure consult service. Ann Pharmacother 2019;53(9):905–15.

13. Ingram A, Valente M, Dzurec MA. Evaluating pharmacist impact on guideline-directed medical therapy in patients with reduced ejection fraction heart failure. J Pharm Pract 2019. 897190019866930.

14. McKinley D, Moye-Dickerson P, Davis S, et al. Impact of a pharmacist-led intervention on 30-day readmission and assessment of factors predictive of readmission in African American men with heart failure. Am J Mens Health 2019;13(1). 1557988318814295.

15. Andersson B, Kjork E, Brunlof G. Temporal improvement in heart failure survival related to the use of a nurse-directed clinic and recommended pharmacological treatment. Int J Cardiol 2005;104(3):257–63.

16. Balakumaran K, Patil A, Marsh S, et al. Evaluation of a guideline directed medical therapy titration program in patients with heart failure with reduced ejection fraction. Int J Cardiol Heart Vasc 2019;22:1–5.

17. O'Connor CM. Guideline-directed medical therapy clinics: a call to action for the heart failure team. JACC Heart Fail 2019;7(5):442–3.

18. Myhre PL, Januzzi JL Jr, Butler J, et al. De novo heart failure: where the journey begins. Eur J Heart Fail 2019;21(10):1245–7.

19. Hong Y, LaBresh KA. Overview of the American Heart Association "Get with the Guidelines" programs: coronary heart disease, stroke, and heart failure. Crit Pathw Cardiol 2006;5(4):179–86.

20. Heidenreich PA, Hernandez AF, Yancy CW, et al. Get with the guidelines program participation, process of care, and outcome for Medicare patients hospitalized with heart failure. Circ Cardiovasc Qual Outcomes 2012;5(1):37–43.

21. Bergethon KE, Ju C, DeVore AD, et al. Trends in 30-day readmission rates for patients hospitalized with heart failure: findings from the get with the guidelines-heart failure registry. Circ Heart Fail 2016;9(6).

22. Fonarow GC, Abraham WT, Albert NM, et al. Organized program to initiate lifesaving treatment in hospitalized patients with heart failure (OPTIMIZE-HF): rationale and design. Am Heart J 2004;148(1): 43–51.

23. Curtis LH, Greiner MA, Hammill BG, et al. Representativeness of a national heart failure quality-of-care registry: comparison of OPTIMIZE-HF and non-OPTIMIZE-HF Medicare patients. Circ Cardiovasc Qual Outcomes 2009;2(4):377–84.

24. Mentz RJ, DeVore A, Tasissa G, et al. Predischarge initiation of ivabradine in the management of heart

failure: results of the PRIME-HF trial. Circ Cardiovasc Qual Outcomes 2019;12:A252.

25. Gattis WA, O'Connor CM, Gallup DS, et al. Predischarge initiation of carvedilol in patients hospitalized for decompensated heart failure: results of the initiation management predischarge: process for Assessment of Carvedilol Therapy in Heart Failure (IMPACT-HF) trial. J Am Coll Cardiol 2004;43(9):1534–41.

26. Velazquez EJ, Morrow DA, DeVore AD, et al. Angiotensin-neprilysin inhibition in acute decompensated heart failure. N Engl J Med 2019;380(6):539–48.

27. Van Spall HGC, Lee SF, Xie F, et al. Effect of patient-centered transitional care services on clinical outcomes in patients hospitalized for heart failure: the PACT-HF randomized clinical trial. JAMA 2019;321(8):753–61.

28. Chaudhry SI, Mattera JA, Curtis JP, et al. Telemonitoring in patients with heart failure. N Engl J Med 2010;363(24):2301–9.

29. Koehler F, Koehler K, Deckwart O, et al. Efficacy of telemedical interventional management in patients with heart failure (TIM-HF2): a randomised, controlled, parallel-group, unmasked trial. Lancet 2018;392(10152):1047–57.

30. Eurlings C, Boyne JJ, de Boer RA, et al. Telemedicine in heart failure-more than nice to have? Neth Heart J 2019;27(1):5–15.

31. Inglis SC, Clark RA, McAlister FA, et al. Structured telephone support or telemonitoring programmes for patients with chronic heart failure. Cochrane Database Syst Rev 2010;(8):CD007228.

32. Werhahn SM, Dathe H, Rottmann T, et al. Designing meaningful outcome parameters using mobile technology: a new mobile application for telemonitoring of patients with heart failure. ESC Heart Fail 2019;6(3):516–25.

33. Givertz MM, Stevenson LW, Costanzo MR, et al. Pulmonary artery pressure-guided management of patients with heart failure and reduced ejection fraction. J Am Coll Cardiol 2017;70(15):1875–86.

34. Abraham WT, Adamson PB, Bourge RC, et al. Wireless pulmonary artery haemodynamic monitoring in chronic heart failure: a randomised controlled trial. Lancet 2011;377(9766):658–66.

35. Sharma A, Zhao X, Hammill BG, et al. Trends in non-cardiovascular comorbidities among patients hospitalized for heart failure: insights from the get with the guidelines-heart failure registry. Circ Heart Fail 2018;11(6):e004646.

36. Guder G, Brenner S, Stork S, et al. Chronic obstructive pulmonary disease in heart failure: accurate diagnosis and treatment. Eur J Heart Fail 2014;16(12):1273–82.

37. Lawson CA, Solis-Trapala I, Dahlstrom U, et al. Comorbidity health pathways in heart failure patients: a sequences-of-regressions analysis using cross-sectional data from 10,575 patients in the Swedish Heart Failure Registry. PLoS Med 2018;15(3):e1002540.

38. Adams KF Jr, Fonarow GC, Emerman CL, et al. Characteristics and outcomes of patients hospitalized for heart failure in the United States: rationale, design, and preliminary observations from the first 100,000 cases in the Acute Decompensated Heart Failure National Registry (ADHERE). Am Heart J 2005;149(2):209–16.

39. O'Connor CM, Abraham WT, Albert NM, et al. Predictors of mortality after discharge in patients hospitalized with heart failure: an analysis from the Organized Program to Initiate Lifesaving Treatment in Hospitalized Patients with Heart Failure (OPTIMIZE-HF). Am Heart J 2008;156(4):662–73.

40. Zinman B, Wanner C, Lachin JM, et al. Empagliflozin, cardiovascular outcomes, and mortality in type 2 diabetes. N Engl J Med 2015;373(22):2117–28.

41. Neal B, Perkovic V, Mahaffey KW, et al. Canagliflozin and cardiovascular and renal events in type 2 diabetes. N Engl J Med 2017;377(7):644–57.

42. Wiviott SD, Raz I, Bonaca MP, et al. Dapagliflozin and cardiovascular outcomes in type 2 diabetes. N Engl J Med 2019;380(4):347–57.

43. Zelniker TA, Braunwald E. Cardiac and renal effects of sodium-glucose co-transporter 2 inhibitors in diabetes: JACC state-of-the-art review. J Am Coll Cardiol 2018;72(15):1845–55.

44. Pasternak B, Ueda P, Eliasson B, et al. Use of sodium glucose cotransporter 2 inhibitors and risk of major cardiovascular events and heart failure: Scandinavian register based cohort study. BMJ 2019;366:l4772.

45. McMurray JJV, Solomon SD, Inzucchi SE, et al. Dapagliflozin in patients with heart failure and reduced ejection fraction. N Engl J Med 2019;381:1995–2008.

46. Canepa M, Temporelli PL, Rossi A, et al. Prevalence and prognostic impact of chronic obstructive pulmonary disease in patients with chronic heart failure: data from the GISSI-HF trial. Cardiology 2017;136(2):128–37.

47. Hawkins NM, Virani S, Ceconi C. Heart failure and chronic obstructive pulmonary disease: the challenges facing physicians and health services. Eur Heart J 2013;34(36):2795–803.

48. Allen LA, Fonarow GC, Liang L, et al. Medication initiation burden required to comply with heart failure guideline recommendations and hospital quality measures. Circulation 2015;132(14):1347–53.

49. Newhouse A, Jiang W. Heart failure and depression. Heart Fail Clin 2014;10(2):295–304.

50. Rutledge T, Reis VA, Linke SE, et al. Depression in heart failure a meta-analytic review of prevalence, intervention effects, and associations with clinical outcomes. J Am Coll Cardiol 2006;48(8):1527–37.

51. Jeyanantham K, Kotecha D, Thanki D, et al. Effects of cognitive behavioural therapy for depression in heart failure patients: a systematic review and meta-analysis. Heart Fail Rev 2017;22(6):731–41.

52. Bhatt AS, DeVore AD, Hernandez AF, et al. Can vaccinations improve heart failure outcomes?: contemporary data and future directions. JACC Heart Fail 2017;5(3):194–203.

53. Udell JA, Zawi R, Bhatt DL, et al. Association between influenza vaccination and cardiovascular outcomes in high-risk patients: a meta-analysis. JAMA 2013;310(16):1711–20.

54. Modin D, Jorgensen ME, Gislason G, et al. Influenza vaccine in heart failure. Circulation 2019;139(5):575–86.

55. Vardeny O, Claggett B, Udell JA, et al. Influenza vaccination in patients with chronic heart failure: the PARADIGM-HF trial. JACC Heart Fail 2016;4(2):152–8.

56. Bhatt AS, Liang L, DeVore AD, et al. Vaccination trends in patients with heart failure: insights from get with the guidelines-heart failure. JACC Heart Fail 2018;6(10):844–55.

57. McKelvie RS. Exercise training in patients with heart failure: clinical outcomes, safety, and indications. Heart Fail Rev 2008;13(1):3–11.

58. O'Connor CM, Whellan DJ, Lee KL, et al. Efficacy and safety of exercise training in patients with chronic heart failure: HF-ACTION randomized controlled trial. JAMA 2009;301(14):1439–50.

59. Mediano MFF, Leifer ES, Cooper LS, et al. Influence of baseline physical activity level on exercise training response and clinical outcomes in heart failure: the HF-ACTION trial. JACC Heart Fail 2018;6(12):1011–9.

60. Chen SM, Fang YN, Wang LY, et al. Impact of multidisciplinary treatment strategy on systolic heart failure outcome. BMC Cardiovasc Disord 2019;19(1):220.

61. Butler T. Dietary management of heart failure: room for improvement? Br J Nutr 2016;115(7):1202–17.

62. Rahman A, Jafry S, Jeejeebhoy K, et al. Malnutrition and cachexia in heart failure. JPEN J Parenter Enteral Nutr 2016;40(4):475–86.

Addressing Comorbidities in Heart Failure
Hypertension, Atrial Fibrillation, and Diabetes

Aakash Bavishi, MD[a], Ravi B. Patel, MD[b],*

KEYWORDS

• Heart failure • Prevalence • Diabetes mellitus • Atrial fibrillation • Hypertension

KEY POINTS

• Hypertension, atrial fibrillation (AF), and diabetes are comorbidities that alter the trajectory of heart failure (HF) and require specialized management.
• Aggressive treatment of hypertension is beneficial in patients with stage A and stage B HF. In stage C HF, hypertension management occurs in parallel with maximization of guideline-directed therapies.
• The management of AF in HF is complex and requires comprehensive evaluation of (1) cause of cardiomyopathy, (2) left ventricular function, (3) symptom burden, and (4) discussion regarding benefits and risks of procedural therapies for AF.
• Novel glucose-lowering therapies have demonstrated particular benefit in the setting of HF. Sodium-glucose cotransporter 2 inhibitors represent a glucose-lowering therapy that has emerged as a cornerstone of therapy in HF with reduced ejection fraction, regardless of diabetes status.

INTRODUCTION

Heart failure (HF) currently affects 6.2 million adults in the United States and is associated with a substantial burden to the health care system, with direct annual cost of $11 billion in 2014.[1,2] Alarmingly, projections indicate that by the year 2030, 8 million people in the United States will have HF, with direct costs expected to surpass 53 billion dollars.[1,3] Similar concerning trends are evident worldwide, as the global prevalence of HF is estimated to be 26 million and increasing.[4] The increasing prevalence of HF cannot be fully attributed to a rising incidence, as HF incidence has remained relatively stable due to substantial improvements in prevention and treatment of acute coronary syndromes.[4–6] An aging population, coupled with advancements in HF management, are likely key contributors to the rising prevalence of HF, as more individuals are now living with HF. Furthermore, there has been a temporal increase in the proportion of patients with heart failure with preserved ejection fraction (HFpEF) as the population ages. Because of growth of the HF population and shift in its makeup to include a higher proportion of elderly individuals with HFpEF, the accumulation of comorbidities is common and represents an additional clinical challenge in providing optimal care in HF. Several comorbidities, including hypertension (HTN), atrial fibrillation (AF), and diabetes mellitus (DM), are not only commonly associated with HF but also may be linked to worse clinical outcomes.[7–9] Thus, optimal management of these comorbidities is

[a] Division of Cardiology, Department of Medicine, Northwestern University Feinberg School of Medicine, Chicago, IL, USA; [b] Division of Cardiology, Department of Medicine, Northwestern University Feinberg School of Medicine, 676 North St Clair Street, Suite 600, Chicago, IL 60611, USA
* Corresponding author.
E-mail address: ravi.patel@northwestern.edu
Twitter: @RBPatelMD (R.B.P.)

Heart Failure Clin 16 (2020) 441–456
https://doi.org/10.1016/j.hfc.2020.06.005
1551-7136/20/© 2020 Elsevier Inc. All rights reserved.

paramount. In this review, the authors describe the HF-specific epidemiology, management strategies, and future directions of research in these 3 disease states.

HYPERTENSION
Epidemiology

According to the 2017 American College of Cardiology/American Heart Association (ACC/AHA) definition, more than 103 million individuals in the United States are burdened with HTN.[10,11] Although the age-standardized prevalence of HTN has decreased, the absolute HTN burden in the United States has increased.[12] In 2010, the global prevalence of HTN was 1.4 billion people with projections that prevalence will exceed 1.6 billion people by 2025.[13]

HTN and HF are inextricably linked. Of 5143 patients in the Framingham Heart Study, HTN preceded the development of HF in 91% of all patients with newly diagnosed HF over the course of 20 years of follow-up.[14,15] Hypertensive men and women are at 2- and 3-fold increased risk of developing HF, respectively, compared with normotensive subjects.[7]

Important racial disparities exist in prevalence and management of HTN. African Americans in the United States are more likely to have HTN compared with other ethnic groups and are less likely to reach target blood pressure goal.[16–18] The disproportionate prevalence of HTN in African Americans is directly associated with higher rates of incident HF in this racial group.[19,20]

Management of Hypertension in Heart Failure

The American College of Cardiology/American Heart Association (ACC/AHA) stage-wide classification of HF includes 4 categories of HF based on the presence or absence of risk factors, structural heart disease, or HF symptoms.[21] Stage A represents those with risk factors for HF, stage B indicates the presence of structural heart disease, stage C represents those with prior or current HF symptoms and stage D indicates refractory HF. This schema is useful to guide HTN management in patients at risk for HF or with prevalent HF. Across all strata of HF, lifestyle counseling regarding diet, weight loss, exercise, smoking cessation, and alcohol moderation is strongly recommended.[22] Current guidelines additionally recommend treatment of blood pressure (BP) to less than 130/80 mm Hg among those at increased risk for HF (stage A) based on the results of Systolic Blood Pressure Intervention Trial (SPRINT), which demonstrated a reduction in incidence of HF among trial participants treated to this

target.[21,23] In general, the optimal blood pressure target for the treatment of HTN in the setting of clinically manifest HF has not been well established. Current guidelines have extended the recommendation of systolic BP less than 130 mm Hg to those patients with stage C HF, regardless of ejection fraction.[21] These recommendations are primarily based on the results of the SPRINT trial, with the acknowledgment that this evidence was not specifically generated from patients with prevalent HF. Detailed approaches to HTN management in HF, including the choice of specific pharmacologic agents, are displayed in **Table 1** and **Fig. 1**. **Table 1** depicts an approach to HTN management based on ACC/AHA stage of HF. A generalized approach to hypertension management in patients with HF is additionally shown in **Fig. 1**.

Future Directions

Further investigation is required to determine the ideal BP target among those patients with stage C HF, regardless of ejection fraction. This is particularly important given the apparent paradox between BP and prognosis once HF with reduced ejection fraction (HFrEF) is present. Specifically, despite the association of BP with incident HF, lower BP is associated with worse prognosis in the setting of overt HFrEF.[24]

In addition, further clarification regarding the utility of specific antihypertensive therapies in preventing HF among those at higher risk is warranted. Indeed, chlorthalidone was associated with reduction in HF risk as compared with amlodipine in the Anti-Hypertensive and Lipid-Lowering Treatment to Prevent Heart Attack (ALLHAT) trial.[25] The antihypertensive effect of sacubitril-valsartan, an angiotensin receptor-neprilysin inhibitor, is stronger than angiotensin receptor blockers (ARBs) or angiotensin-converting enzyme inhibitors alone and thus increases the possibility that this agent may also be particularly effective in curbing HF risk among those at high risk.

Regardless of the approach, it is becoming increasingly clear that a team-based, collaborative effort to managing HTN is of benefit to the patient with HF.[26] Collaboration between nephrologists, cardiologists, and internists to create a personalized treatment strategy to which patients can easily adhere is critical. Collaboration between physicians, pharmacists, midlevel providers, and social workers is essential to create more opportunities for lifestyle and medication interventions, and address economic and social barriers to care. Several technological innovations such as

Table 1
Management of hypertension by American College of Cardiology/American Heart Association stage of heart failure

Stage A HF	Stage B HF	Stage C HF

• Heart healthy lifestyle
• Aggressive BP management
  ○ Target BP <130/80 to reduce risk of overt HF[14]
• Choosing specific agent
  ○ Chlorthalidone is associated with reduced HF risk compared with amlodipine or lisinopril[87]
  ○ Calcium-channel blockers, thiazide diuretics, ACE-I, or ARB are appropriate first-line agents[88]
  ○ In diabetic patients with nephropathy, ARB have been shown to be efficacious in reducing incident HF risk[89]
• Secondary HTN workup in patients with persistent HTN
  ○ Including OSA screening[90]
	• In patients with LV dysfunction, there is robust data supporting the use of ACE-I and β blockers in promoting LV recovery[94–97]
	• Although these LV benefits are not exclusive to the HTN population, many patients with LV dysfunction also have HTN
	• Avoidance of nondihydropyridine calcium channel blockers and alpha-adrenergic blockers[25]
		• Heart healthy lifestyle
		• Systolic BP goal <130 mm Hg
		• Heart failure with reduced ejection fraction
		  ○ Optimization of β blocker, ACE-I/ARB or ARNI, and MRA to target levels
		  ○ ARNI in particular has potent antihypertensive effects[25]
		  ○ Most patients are not appropriately uptitrated to target doses despite significant room in their BP[91,92]
		• Heart Failure with preserved ejection fraction
		  ○ Consider MRA to reduce HF hospitalization
		  ○ Consider ARNI in select subgroups (ie, women, mid-range EF)
		• Diuretics
		  ○ Loop diuretics have minimal antihypertensive effects compared with thiazide diuretics[93]
		  ○ Thiazide diuretics can be considered in patients with minimal congestive symptoms and persistently high BP
		• Secondary HTN workup in patients with persistent HTN, including OSA screening[90]

Abbreviations: ACE-I, angiotensin-converting enzyme inhibitor; ARB, angiotensin receptor blocker; ARNI, angiotensin receptor-neprilysin inhibitor; LV, left ventricular; MRA, mineralocorticoid receptor antagonist; OSA, obstructive sleep apnea.

text message reminders and mobile app notifications have shown promise in improving medication adherence and may have an important role in the comprehensive treatment plan for hypertensive patients.[27–29] In addition, HTN management is based on the same principle as guideline-directed medical therapy in HFrEF: the timely initiation and titration of pharmacotherapy to goal doses. As such, frequent visits with various members of the medical team, including HF nurse practitioners, may be particularly important to reach target BP goals in HF.

ATRIAL FIBRILLATION
Epidemiology

Current estimations demonstrate that between 2.7 and 6.1 million people in the United States have AF and more than 33.5 million individuals worldwide are burdened by AF.[10,30] There has been a consistent increase in the incidence and prevalence of AF, as AF is predicted to affect 6 to 12 million people in the United States by 2050 and 17.9 million in Europe by 2060.[30–34] The increased incidence and prevalence have been attributed to both increases in prevalence of risk factors for AF (ie, DM and obesity) as well as the heightened awareness and detection of AF.[31,35,36]

Up to 62% of individuals with HF may have AF at some point during their life course.[37] Indeed, AF and HF share several common, underlying risk factors. There seems to be a bidirectional relationship between these 2 disease states, in which each disease induces inflammatory, neurohormonal, and structural changes that predisposes to the other syndrome.[38] In addition, numerous studies have demonstrated that patients with both AF and HF have worse short-term and long-term outcomes than either condition alone.[8,39–41]

Management of Atrial Fibrillation in Patients with Heart Failure

The approach to management of AF in patients with HF depends on several factors, including the acuity of each condition, degree of HF decompensation, left ventricular function, and presence of other structural heart abnormalities (**Fig. 2**).

In the setting of acute decompensated HF with concomitant AF and rapid ventricular rate, primary clinical goals should be decongestion and consideration of agents to carefully lower ventricular rate. Caution should be taken in aggressive rate control in the setting of acute HF, as patients with significantly decompensated HF may not tolerate a sudden decrement in ventricular rate. In patients with HFrEF, nondihydropyridine calcium channel blockers should be avoided. Amiodarone and

digoxin may be appropriate therapies in the acute setting until patients are decongested and can tolerate titration of β blocker therapy. In patients with HFpEF, nondihydropyridine calcium channel blockers or β blockers may be useful to acutely control heart rate. If AF is determined to be the true trigger for HF decompensation, an acute rhythm control strategy can also be pursued. The optimal timing of rhythm control of AF via cardioversion during the course of hospitalization for HF is not well understood.

In the nonacute setting, the decision whether to pursue a rate or rhythm control strategy is multifaceted and should be based on careful discussions with patients regarding risks and benefits, along with assessment of ejection fraction (see **Fig. 2**). Symptomatic AF may influence the decision to pursue a rhythm controlling strategy in the setting of HF. However, the degree to which AF contributes to symptoms such as dyspnea or fatigue in patients with HF and AF is especially challenging. First, the constellation of symptoms in AF and HF is overlapping and may be difficult to distinguish. Indeed, dyspnea and nonspecific fatigue are hallmarks of both syndromes. In addition, inactive lifestyle and functional limitations due to HF may mask symptomatic AF, which may only be manifest at higher ventricular rates.

There is limited efficacy of antiarrhythmic drug (AAD) therapy for rhythm control in the setting of AF and HF. The Atrial Fibrillation and Congestive Heart Failure (AF-CHF) trial did not demonstrate a significant reduction in cardiovascular mortality with rhythm control compared with rate control among patients with HFrEF.[42] In addition, the Danish Investigators of Arrhythmia Mortality on Dofetilide in Congestive Heart Failure (DIAMOND-CHF) trial, which compared dofetilide with placebo in HFrEF, failed to show an improvement in mortality. However, a reduction in hospitalizations was noted in the dofetilide arm in DIAMOND-CHF.[43]

The limited efficacy of AAD led to speculation that maintenance of sinus rhythm through catheter ablation (CA) may be more beneficial to patients with HF compared with AAD alone. In HFrEF, several small studies have shown improvement in exercise capacity, quality-of-life metrics, and left ventricular function with CA, although data regarding clinical cardiovascular outcomes are limited.[44–48] A small multicenter randomized study showed the superior efficacy of CA compared with amiodarone in reducing unplanned hospitalizations and mortality in patients with HFrEF.[49] Subsequently, results from the recent Catheter Ablation versus Standard Conventional Therapy

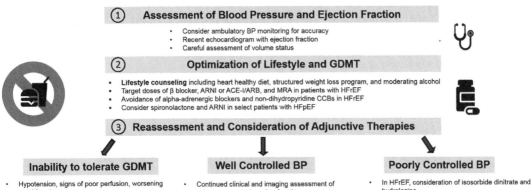

Fig. 1. Hypertension management in established heart failure. ACE-I, angiotensin converting enzyme inhibitors; ARB, angiotensin receptor blocker; ARNI, angiotensin receptor-neprilysin inhibitor; BP, blood pressure; CCBs, calcium channel blocker; GDMT, guideline-directed medical therapy; HF, heart failure; HFpEF, heart failure with preserved ejection fraction; HFrEF, heart failure with reduced ejection fraction; MRA, mineralocorticoid receptor antagonist; OSA, obstructive sleep apnea.

in Patients with Left Ventricular Dysfunction and Atrial Fibrillation (CASTLE-AF) trial demonstrated that in patients with AF and symptomatic HFrEF (left ventricular ejection fraction [LVEF] ≤35%), CA was associated with a significant reduction in death and hospitalization for HF, greater improvement in LVEF, and long-term maintenance of sinus rhythm.[50] Significant questions remain about generalizability of CASTLE-AF findings, given the highly selected patient population and exclusion of those patients who easily achieved rhythm control.[50] The results of this study were reflected in the 2019 update to the 2014 AHA/ACC/Heart Rhythm Society Guidelines for AF management, which stated that CA may be reasonable in selected patients with HFrEF to potentially lower mortality rate and reduce hospitalization for HF (class IIB recommendation).[51]

Despite the prevalence and significant adverse effects of AF in HFpEF, data are even more limited with regard to management of AF in this vulnerable population.[52,53] Aggressive management of obstructive sleep apnea, obesity, and DM should be pursued, which has been shown to reduce AF recurrence and improve cardiorespiratory fitness in HFpEF.[54–57] Observational studies have demonstrated associations of rhythm control of AF with improved quality of life, functional capacity, and lower all-cause mortality in HFpEF.[58,59] However, randomized clinical trial evidence is currently lacking. Similar to management of AF in all patients with HF, a comprehensive patient-specific evaluation—including careful symptom assessment,

cardiac monitoring to assess efficacy of rate control, and patient preference—is needed to determine AF treatment strategy. In specific patient populations, such as restrictive cardiomyopathy or hypertrophic cardiomyopathy in which the atrial contractile function is critical to hemodynamics, aggressive strategies for rhythm control should be pursued. In patients whom AF is thought to be driving frequent HF hospitalizations, a more aggressive rhythm control strategy should be pursued.

Finally, in the absence of compelling contraindications, all patients should be anticoagulated regardless of LVEF.[60] Multiple large meta-analyses have confirmed the efficacy and safety of non-vitamin K antagonist oral anticoagulants in patients with AF and HF.[61,62]

Because of current gaps in evidence, there is no widely accepted treatment pathway for the management of AF in HF. As such, the authors provide a general approach to comprehensive management of AF in HF in **Fig. 2**.

Future Directions

Significant research is still needed to define optimal AF management strategies in HF. In the setting of HFrEF, additional clinical trials of CA, inclusive of broader populations and of larger sample size, are necessary to confirm the suggested benefits of CA noted in the CASTLE-AF trial. Identification of patients with HFrEF who are most likely to benefit from upfront CA without an initial

Comprehensive, Personalized Assessment of AF

- Ensure accurate documentation of AF
- Assess AF burden and rate control
- Evaluation of patient symptoms and correlation with AF
- Consideration of patient-specific pathology (LVEF, nature of cardiomyopathy, cardiac and non-cardiac comorbidities)
- Understanding of patient preference and values
- **Lifestyle counseling**: encourage weight loss, ensure strict control of HTN and DM, and screen for OSA

② **Choose Initial Rate or Rhythm Control Strategy**

Factors favoring Rate Control
- Failure of rhythm control
- Patient preference
- Limited correlation between AF and HF symptoms and hospitalizations

Factors favoring Rhythm Control
- Failure of rate control
- Repeat HF hospitalizations with AF as trigger
- Symptomatic AF
- Patient preference

Treatment Options
- β blockers 1st line in HFrEF
- Avoidance of non-dihydropyridine CCBs in HFrEF
- Frequent reassessment of efficacy of rate control strategy (may require monitoring)
- Consider AV nodal ablation with PPM or CRT-P in refractory cases

Treatment Options
- Consider CA as first line in select HFrEF patients to reduce hospitalizations/mortality
- After DCCV or CA, consider maintenance AAD including dofetilide, amiodarone, or sotalol
- Avoidance of dronedarone in HFrEF and Class IC agents in all HF
- CA in symptomatic HF patients after failed AAD

 Anticoagulation unless contraindications

Fig. 2. Atrial fibrillation management in chronic heart failure. AAD, antiarrhythmic drug; AF, atrial fibrillation; AV, atrioventricular; CA, catheter ablation; CCBs, calcium channel blocker; CRT-P, cardiac resynchronization therapy pacemaker; DCCV, direct current cardioversion; DM, diabetes mellitus; HF, heart failure; HFpEF, heart failure with preserved ejection fraction; HFrEF, heart failure with reduced ejection fraction; HTN, hypertension; LVEF, left ventricular ejection fraction; OSA, obstructive sleep apnea; PPM, permanent pacemaker.

trial of AAD therapy may also be important to further understand.

There is currently a lack of evidence for CA in the setting of HFpEF. Although an intention to treat analysis of the recent Catheter Ablation vs Antiarrhythmic Drug Therapy for Atrial Fibrillation (CABANA) trial demonstrated a decrease in mortality, stroke, and cardiac arrest in patients with HF undergoing CA compared with medical therapy (rate or rhythm control), characterization of HF by ejection fraction status was not fully captured in this analysis.[63] Given the frequent coexistence of AF and HFpEF and the association of AF with worse long-term outcomes, trial-level evidence for treatment of AF in HFpEF represents a critical unmet need.

Further research is also needed to identify which patients would benefit from CA compared with invasive rate control through atrioventricular (AV)

nodal ablation with pacing. The Pulmonary Vein Antrum Isolation vs AV Node Ablation with Bi-Ventricular Pacing for Treatment of Atrial Fibrillation in Patients with Congestive Heart Failure demonstrated improvement in quality of life, LV function, and 6-minute walk test at 6 months in patients undergoing pulmonary vein isolation compared with patients undergoing AV nodal ablation with biventricular pacing.[64] However, this study was limited in sample size and duration (6 months). The effect of AV nodal ablation and pacing compared with CA is being further investigated in the Rhythm Control-Catheter Ablation With or Without Antiarrhythmic Drug Control of Maintaining Sinus Rhythm vs Rate Control with Medical Therapy and/or Atrio-ventricular Junction Ablation and Pacemaker Treatment for Atrial Fibrillation (RAFT-AF) clinical trial (NCT01420393), which will include patients with both HFrEF and

HFpEF with New York Heart Association class II or III symptoms.

DIABETES MELLITUS
Epidemiology

In recent decades, the prevalence of DM has increased both globally and within the United States. Worldwide, the prevalence of DM increased from 180 million in 1980 to 422 million in October 2014.[65] There were 30.3 million Americans with diabetes in 2015, and 2030 projections estimate 54.9 million Americans will have DM with total costs expected to surpass $622 billion.[66,67] Given the relatively stable incidence, the increasing prevalence of DM is due to a combination of an aging population, increase in obesity, dramatic increase in DM cases in children and adolescents, and improved medical care prolonging life in diabetic patients.[67]

DM and HF commonly coexist, as rates of DM are as high as 47% in HF cohorts.[68–71] Individuals with DM are at a 2 to 4 times increased risk of developing HF, with higher risks in women and younger adults.[68,72] Several mechanisms underlie the increased HF risk in patients with DM, including (1) myocardial ischemia and infarction in setting of accelerated atherosclerosis; (2) fibrosis with myocardial stiffness due to advanced glycosylation end products; (3) oxidative stress; (4) autonomic dysfunction; (5) upregulation of the renin-angiotensin system; and (6) defects at cardiomyocyte level in contraction and relaxation.[73] Patients with HF who have DM have more frequent HF hospitalizations, lower quality of life, and higher mortality than patients with HF without DM.[9,74–76]

Management of Diabetes Mellitus in Heart Failure

Because the 2008 Food and Drug Administration mandate that cardiovascular safety be established among all new glucose lowering therapies, there have been numerous, large-scale clinical trials evaluating the effect of various antidiabetic drugs on cardiovascular outcomes. This inundation of outcomes trials has revealed important insights into specific cardiovascular benefits of certain glucose-lowering therapies in the setting of HF. A summary of antihyperglycemic agents and their impact on HF outcomes is shown in **Table 2**. The aggregate data have demonstrated a consistent benefit of sodium-glucose cotransporter 2 (SGLT2) inhibitors in reducing HF hospitalizations among patients with diabetes at moderate-to-high baseline cardiovascular risk. Although another class of drugs, glucagon-like peptide-1 receptor agonists, has also demonstrated

cardiovascular risk reduction, such effects do not seem to be driven by a reduction in HF events. More recently, a specific SGLT2 inhibitor, dapagliflozin, demonstrated substantial reductions in cardiovascular mortality and HF hospitalizations among those with HFrEF regardless of diabetes status in the Dapagliflozin and Prevention of Adverse Outcomes in Heart Failure (DAPA-HF) trial.[77] As such, SGLT2 inhibitors will likely represent the newest disease-modifying therapy in HFrEF. In the setting of HFrEF in particular, this drug class should be considered a first-line therapy, regardless of diabetes status.

Among diabetic patients at risk for HF, the first-line glucose-lowering therapy is currently controversial. Given the consistent benefit of SGLT2 inhibitors in reducing cardiovascular mortality or HF hospitalization in this population, some medical societies have recommended concurrent consideration of SGLT2 inhibitors with metformin initiation.[78] Currently, according to the American Diabetes Association, metformin is still considered the first-line diabetic regimen in all patients and has been proved to be safe in patients with HF without significant chronic kidney disease.[79]

In patients with HF, we have proposed an algorithm for selection of glucose-lowering therapies (**Fig. 3**). Several factors must be accounted for when selecting proper antihyperglycemic agents for patients with HF, including kidney function, medication interactions, burden of polypharmacy, risk of hypoglycemia, and concurrent cardiac and noncardiac comorbidities (see **Table 2**). In general, given the signal of benefit from the SGLT2 inhibitor class across major cardiovascular outcome trials in reducing HF hospitalizations, we favor timely initiation of this therapeutic class, regardless of ejection fraction.

Of note, there is no current data supporting intensive hyperglycemic control in patients with DM to reduce risk of incident HF.[80] The association between HbA_{1C} and HF mortality is generally U-shaped, with a nadir of risk at HbA_{1C} 7% to 8%.[81,82] Indeed, HbA_{1C} reductions in large-scale outcomes trials of antidiabetic drugs have been modest, and HF benefits are in general felt to be independent of degree of HbA_{1c} reduction.[70]

Future Directions

The dogma that metformin is the foundational, first therapy for all diabetics may come under scrutiny in the future. Indeed, in HFrEF, one may argue that SGLT2 inhibitors should be the first-line therapy for cardiovascular risk reduction in light of the DAPA-HF trial. Across the spectrum of new diabetes, the efficacy of metformin as a first-line

Table 2
Impact of glucose-lowering therapies on heart failure outcomes: a summary of randomized clinical trials

	Mechanism	Key RCTs	HF Specific Data	Disadvantages
Metformin	Decreases hepatic glucose production Decreases intestinal absorption of glucose Increases insulin sensitivity	None	Safe in patients with HF[98]	Nausea, abdominal discomfort
Sulfonylureas	Closure of ATP-sensitive potassium channels to stimulate insulin release from β-cells	CAROLINA: noninferiority trial of linagliptin vs glimepiride in patients with DM with elevated CV risk[99]	No difference in HF hospitalization with glimepiride compared with linagliptin[99]	Hypoglycemia, weight gain
Meglitinides	Closure of ATP-sensitive potassium channels to stimulate insulin release from β cells	NAVIGATOR: 9306 participants with impaired fasting glucose randomized to nateglinide or placebo[100]	No difference in HF hospitalization with nateglinide: HR = 0.85 (95% CI: 0.64–1.14)	
α-Glucosidase inhibitors	Delay carbohydrate digestion; reduces rate of intestinal glucose absorption	ACE: 6522 patients with impaired glucose tolerance and CAD randomized to acarbose or placebo[101]	No difference in HF hospitalization: HR = 0.89 (95% CI: 0.63–1.24)	
Insulin	Several mechanisms leading to direct and indirect uptake of glucose in cells	ORIGIN: randomized 12,537 patients with DM or pre-DM w ith CV risk factors to standard of care or insulin glargine[102]	No difference in HF hospitalization with insulin glargine compared with standard of care: HR = 0.90, (95% CI: 0.77–1.05)[102]	Cost; Hypoglycemia
Thiazolidinediones	Activating PPAR nuclear receptors leads to upregulation of genes resulting in decreased insulin resistance	PROACTIVE: 5238 patients with DM and macrovascular disease randomized to pioglitazone or placebo[103] RECORD: 4447 patients with DM on metformin or sulfonylurea monotherapy randomized to addition of rosiglitazone or combination of metformin or sulfonylurea[104]	Increased risk of HF admission[103] Increased risk of HF causing hospitalization or death with rosiglitazone: HR = 2.1 (95% CI: 1.35–3.27)[104]	Edema, reduction of bone mineral density, increased HF hospitalizations
GLP-1 receptor agonists	Stimulates GLP-1 receptors, thereby increasing insulin secretion and improving insulin sensitivity	Lixisenatide — ELIXA: 6068 patients with DM and ACS randomized to lixisenatide or placebo[105] Liraglutide — LEADER: 9340 patients with DM, high CV risk to receive liraglutide or placebo[106] Semaglutide — SUSTAIN-6: 3297 patients with DM randomized to	No difference in HF hospitalization: HR = 0.96, (95% CI: 0.75–1.23)[105] No difference in HF hospitalization: HR = 0.87, (95% CI: 0.73–1.05)[106] No difference in HF hospitalization:	GI upset, headache

Class	Mechanism	Agent	Trial	Outcome	Adverse effects
			semaglutide or placebo[107]	HR = 1.11, (95% CI: 0.77–1.61) P = .57[107]	
			PIONEER 6: 3182 patients randomized to oral semaglutide vs placebo in DM (noninferiority trial)	No difference in HF hospitalization: HR = 0.86 (95% CI: 0.48–1.55)	
			SOUL: oral semaglutide vs placebo in DM (superiority trial)	Trial Ongoing	
		Exenatide	EXSCEL: 14,752 patients with DM ± CAD were randomized to exenatide or placebo[108]	No difference in HF hospitalization: HR = 0.94, (95% CI: 0.78–1.13)[108]	
		Albiglutide	HARMONY OUTCOMES: 9463 patients with DM and CVD randomized to albiglutide or placebo[109]	No difference in composite of CV death or HF hospitalization: HR = 0.85 (95% CI: 0.70–1.04)	
		Dulaglutide	REWIND: 9901 patients with DM randomized to dulaglutide or placebo	No difference in HF hospitalization: HR = 0.93 (95% CI: 0.77–1.12)	
DPP-4 inhibitors	Slows the inactivation and degradation of GLP-1	Saxagliptin	SAVOR TIMI-53: 16,492 patients with DM with history or at high risk of CVD were randomized to saxagliptin or placebo[110]	Increased rate of HF hospitalization: HR = 1.27, (95% CI: 1.07–1.51)[110]	GI problems, flulike symptoms
		Alogliptin	EXAMINE: 5380 patients with DM and ACS within 90 d to alogliptin or placebo[111]	No difference in HF hospitalization: HR = 1.07, (95% CI: 0.79–1.46)[112]	
		Sitagliptin	TECOS: 14,671 patients with DM and established CVD were assigned to sitagliptin or placebo[113]	No differences in rates of hospitalization for HF: HR = 1.00, (95% CI: 0.83–1.20)[113]	
		Linagliptin	CAROLINA: noninferiority trial of linagliptin vs glimepiride in patients with DM with elevated CV risk[99]	No difference in HF hospitalization with linagliptin compared with glimepiride	
SGLT-2 inhibitors	Inhibits SGLT-2 in proximal-convoluted tubule to prevent reabsorption of glucose and sodium	Empagliflozin	EMPA-REG OUTCOME: 7020 patients with established CVD randomized to empagliflozin or placebo[114]	Reduction in HF hospitalization: HR = 0.65, (95% CI: 0.50–0.85)[114]	Genital yeast infections, urinary tract infections, increased urination, dehydration, constipation

(continued on next page)

Table 2
(continued)

Mechanism	Key RCTs	HF Specific Data	Disadvantages
	EMPEROR-REDUCED: empagliflozin or placebo in HFrEF	*Trial ongoing*	
	EMPEROR-PRESERVED: empagliflozin or placebo in HFpEF	*Trial ongoing*	
	EMPULSE HF: empagliflozin vs placebo in acute hospitalized HF	*Trial ongoing*	
Canagliflozin	CANVAS: 10,142 patients with DM and high CV risk assigned to canagliflozin or placebo[115]	Reduction in HF hospitalization: HR = 0.67 (95% CI: 0.52–0.87)[115]	
	CHIEF-HF: 1900 patients with HF randomized to canagliflozin or placebo	*Trial ongoing*	
Dapagliflozin	DECLARE-TIMI 58: 17,160 patients with DM with or at risk for CVD randomized to dapagliflozin or placebo[116]	Reduction in HF hospitalization: HR = 0.73 (0.61–0.88)[116]	
	DAPA-HF: 4744 patients with NYHA class II–IV HFrEF randomized to dapagliflozin or placebo[77]	Reduction in CV mortality or worsening HF regardless of DM status: HR = 0.74 (95% CI: 0.65–0.85)	
	DELIVER: dapagliflozin vs placebo in HFpEF	*Trial ongoing*	
	DAPA ACT HF-TIMI 68: dapagliflozin vs. placebo in HFrEF after admission for acute HF	*Trial ongoing*	
Sotagliflozin[a]	SOLOIST-WHF: sotaglifozin vs placebo in HFrEF after admission for worsening HF	*Trial ongoing*	
Ertugliflozin	VERTIS CV: ertugliflozin vs placebo in DM with CVD	Reduction in HF hospitalization (2.5% vs. 3.6%); full publication of results forthcoming	

Abbreviations: ACS, acute coronary syndrome; ATP, adenosine triphosphate; CAD, coronary artery disease; CV, cardiovascular; CVD, cardiovascular disease; GI, gastrointestinal; GLP-1 RA, glucagon-like peptide-1; SGLT2, sodium glucose transporter 2.

[a] Combined SGLT-1/SGLT-2 inhibitor.

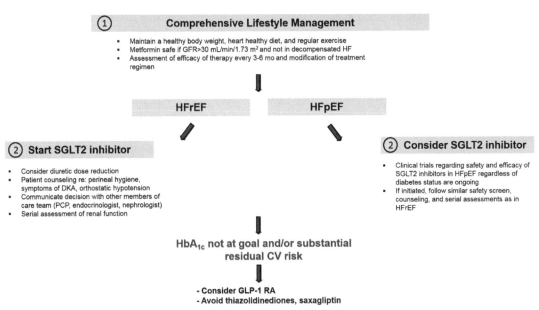

Fig. 3. Diabetes management in chronic heart failure. CV, cardiovascular; DKA, diabetic ketoacidosis; GFR, glomerular filtration rate; GLP-1 RA, glucagon-like peptide-1 receptor agonist; HbA$_{1c}$, hemoglobin A$_{1c}$; HF, heart failure; HFpEF, heart failure with preserved ejection fraction; HFrEF, heart failure with reduced ejection fraction; PCP, primary care physician; SGLT2, sodium glucose transporter 2.

therapy will be evaluated in the SGLT2 Inhibitor or Metformin as Standard Treatment of Early Stage Type 2 Diabetes (SMARTEST) trial, which will randomize more than 4000 new diabetics to metformin or dapagliflozin (NCT03982381).

The efficacy of SGLT2 inhibitors in reducing cardiovascular outcomes in the setting of HFpEF is currently being evaluated in several randomized clinical trials (NCT03057951; NCT03619213; NCT03030235). Given the natriuretic effect of SGLT2 inhibitors and robust clinical benefit of dapagliflozin in HFrEF, there remains substantial promise of this therapeutic class in the HFpEF cohort.

The growing burden of DM and associated high rates of cardiovascular comorbidities highlights the necessity of a comprehensive, multispecialty team, which is inclusive of cardiologists, to address diabetes care. Despite the growing evidence of SGLT2 inhibitors and GLP-1 RA as cardiovascular risk-reducing agents, approximately 90% of diabetes care is restricted to primary care physicians and endocrinologists.[83,84] However, access to endocrinologists for diabetes lags behind access to cardiologists, with disparities especially prominent in certain geographic regions.[85] Indeed, patients with diabetes at high cardiovascular risk encounter cardiologists far more frequently than endocrinologists.[86] Given the density of cardiologists and frequency of cardiology encounters, it is imperative that cardiologists take a more active role in the management of DM, including the prescription of new evidence-based glucose-lowering therapies. Such involvement by cardiologists requires familiarity with drug dosing, side effects, and appropriate patient counseling. Importantly, close communication between all members of the patient's care team, including primary care physician, endocrinologist, nephrologist, and cardiologist, is important to inform appropriate and safe diabetes treatment plans.

SUMMARY

HF represents a growing burden on health care systems in the United States and worldwide. In this review, the authors address 3 comorbidities inextricably associated with HF: HTN, AF, and DM. Timely identification and management of these 3 comorbidities are paramount across the spectrum of HF, from stage A HF to end-stage cardiomyopathy. Because of the aging HF population and increasing proportion of patients with HFpEF, management of HF comorbidities is increasingly complex. However, comorbidity management remains integral in optimizing long-term outcomes. Comorbidity management in HF requires close collaboration between providers and formulation of therapeutic plans that are consistent with patient values and preferences. Although excitement behind new therapeutics is warranted, implementation of lifestyle modifications and relief of socioeconomic barriers to health care remain a critical point of emphasis for physicians. Through concerted efforts across these mechanisms, co-morbidity management has promise in further improving quality of life and clinical outcomes in chronic HF.

DISCLOSURE

Dr A. Bavishi has nothing to disclose. Dr R.B. Patel is supported by the NHLBI T32 postdoctoral training grant (T32HL069771).

REFERENCES

1. Heidenreich PA, Albert NM, Allen LA, et al. Fore-casting the impact of heart failure in the United States. Circ Heart Fail 2013;6(3):606–19.
2. Jackson SL, Tong X, King RJ, et al. National Burden of Heart Failure Events in the United States, 2006 to 2014. Circ Heart Fail 2018;11(12):e004873.
3. Benjamin EJ, Muntner P, Alonso A, et al. Heart dis-ease and stroke statistics-2019 update: a report From the American Heart Association. Circulation 2019;139(10):e56–528.
4. Savarese G, Lund LH. Global Public Health Burden of Heart Failure. Card Fail Rev 2017;3(1):7–11.
5. Levy D, Kenchaiah S, Larson MG, et al. Long-term trends in the incidence of and survival with heart failure. N Engl J Med 2002;347(18):1397–402.
6. Najafi F, Jamrozik K, Dobson AJ. Understanding the 'epidemic of heart failure': a systematic review of trends in determinants of heart failure. Eur J Heart Fail 2009;11(5):472–9.
7. Butler J, Kalogeropoulos AP, Georgiopoulou VV, et al. Systolic blood pressure and incident heart failure in the elderly. The Cardiovascular Health Study and the Health, Ageing and Body Composi-tion Study. Heart 2011;97(16):1304–11.
8. Khazanie P, Liang L, Qualls LG, et al. Outcomes of medicare beneficiaries with heart failure and atrial fibrillation. JACC Heart Fail 2014;2(1):41–8.
9. Allen LA, Gheorghiade M, Reid KJ, et al. Identifying patients hospitalized with heart failure at risk for un-favorable future quality of life. Circ Cardiovasc Qual Outcomes 2011;4(4):389–98.
10. Benjamin EJ, Virani SS, Callaway CW, et al. Heart disease and stroke statistics-2018 update: a report from the American Heart Association. Circulation 2018;137(12):e67.
11. Muntner P, Carey RM, Gidding S, et al. Potential US population impact of the 2017 ACC/AHA high blood pressure guideline. Circulation 2018;137(2):109–18.
12. Dorans KS, Mills KT, Liu Y, et al. Trends in preva-lence and control of hypertension according to the 2017 American College of Cardiology/Amer-ican Heart Association (ACC/AHA) guideline. J Am Heart Assoc 2018;7(11):e008888.
13. Mills KT, Bundy JD, Kelly TN, et al. Global dispar-ities of hypertension prevalence and control: a sys-tematic analysis of population-based studies from 90 countries. Circulation 2016;134(6):441–50.
14. Levy D, Larson MG, Vasan RS, et al. The progres-sion from hypertension to congestive heart failure. JAMA 1996;275(20):1557–62.
15. Messerli FH, Rimoldi SF, Bangalore S. The transi-tion from hypertension to heart failure: contempo-rary update. JACC Heart Fail 2017;5(8):543–51.
16. Hertz RP, Unger AN, Cornell JA, et al. Racial dis-parities in hypertension prevalence, awareness, and management. Arch Intern Med 2005;165(18):2098–104.
17. Yoon SS, Carroll MD, Fryar CD. Hypertension Prev-alence and Control Among Adults: United States, 2011-2014. NCHS Data Brief 2015;(220):1–8.
18. Lackland DT. Racial differences in hypertension: implications for high blood pressure management. Am J Med Sci 2014;348(2):135–8.
19. Bahrami H, Kronmal R, Bluemke DA, et al. Differ-ences in the incidence of congestive heart failure by ethnicity: the multi-ethnic study of atheroscle-rosis. Arch Intern Med 2008;168(19):2138–45.
20. Bibbins-Domingo K, Pletcher MJ, Lin F, et al. Racial differences in incident heart failure among young adults. N Engl J Med 2009;360(12):1179–90.
21. Yancy CW, Jessup M, Bozkurt B, et al. 2017 ACC/AHA/HFSA focused update of the 2013 ACCF/AHA guideline for the management of heart failure: a report of the American College of Cardiology/Amer-ican Heart Association Task Force on Clinical Prac-tice Guidelines and the Heart Failure Society of America. J Am Coll Cardiol 2017;70(6):776–803.
22. Aggarwal M, Bozkurt B, Panjrath G, et al. Lifestyle modifications for preventing and treating heart fail-ure. J Am Coll Cardiol 2018;72(19):2391–405.
23. SPRINT Research Group, Wright JT Jr, Williamson JD, Whelton PK, et al. A randomized trial of intensive versus standard blood-pressure control. N Engl J Med 2015;373(22):2103–16.
24. Ather S, Chan W, Chillar A, et al. Association of sys-tolic blood pressure with mortality in patients with heart failure with reduced ejection fraction: a com-plex relationship. Am Heart J 2011;161(3):567–73.
25. ALLHAT Officers and Coordinators for the ALLHAT Collaborative Research Group. The Antihyperten-sive and Lipid-Lowering Treatment to Prevent Heart Attack Trial. Major outcomes in high-risk hyperten-sive patients randomized to angiotensin-converting enzyme inhibitor or calcium channel blocker vs diuretic: The Antihypertensive and Lipid-Lowering Treatment to Prevent Heart Attack Trial (ALLHAT). JAMA 2002;288(23):2981–97.

26. Proia KK, Thota AB, Njie GJ, et al. Team-based care and improved blood pressure control: a community guide systematic review. Am J Prev Med 2014;47(1):86–99.

27. Kiselev AR, Gridnev VI, Shvartz VA, et al. Active ambulatory care management supported by short message services and mobile phone technology in patients with arterial hypertension. J Am Soc Hypertens 2012;6(5):346–55.

28. Patel S, Jacobus-Kantor L, Marshall L, et al. Mobilizing your medications: an automated medication reminder application for mobile phones and hypertension medication adherence in a high-risk urban population. J Diabetes Sci Technol 2013;7(3): 630–9.

29. Varleta P, Acevedo M, Akel C, et al. Mobile phone text messaging improves antihypertensive drug adherence in the community. J Clin Hypertens 2017;19(12):1276–84.

30. Chugh SS, Havmoeller R, Narayanan K, et al. Worldwide epidemiology of atrial fibrillation: a Global Burden of Disease 2010 Study. Circulation 2014;129(8):837–47.

31. Lane DA, Skjøth F, Lip GY, et al. Temporal trends in incidence, prevalence, and mortality of atrial fibrillation in primary care. J Am Heart Assoc 2017; 6(5):e005155.

32. Lloyd-Jones DM, Wang TJ, Leip EP, et al. Lifetime risk for development of atrial fibrillation: the Framingham Heart Study. Circulation 2004;110(9): 1042–6.

33. Krijthe BP, Kunst A, Benjamin EJ, et al. Projections on the number of individuals with atrial fibrillation in the European Union, from 2000 to 2060. Eur Heart J 2013;34(35):2746–51.

34. Morillo CA, Banerjee A, Perel P, et al. Atrial fibrillation: the current epidemic. J Geriatr Cardiol 2017; 14(3):195–203.

35. Lowres N, Neubeck L, Redfern J, et al. Screening to identify unknown atrial fibrillation. Thromb Haemost 2013;110(08):213–22.

36. Schnabel RB, Yin X, Gona P, et al. 50 year trends in atrial fibrillation prevalence, incidence, risk factors, and mortality in the Framingham Heart Study: a cohort study. Lancet 2015;386(9989): 154–62.

37. Santhanakrishnan R, Wang N, Larson MG, et al. Atrial fibrillation begets heart failure and vice versa: temporal associations and differences in preserved versus reduced ejection fraction. Circulation 2016;133(5):484–92.

38. Batul SA, Gopinathannair R. Atrial fibrillation in heart failure: a therapeutic challenge of our times. Korean Circ J 2017;47(5):644–62.

39. Ling LH, Kistler PM, Kalman JM, et al. Comorbidity of atrial fibrillation and heart failure. Nat Rev Cardiol 2016;13(3):131–47.

40. Wang TJ, Larson MG, Levy D, et al. Temporal relations of atrial fibrillation and congestive heart failure and their joint influence on mortality: the Framingham Heart Study. Circulation 2003;107(23):2920–5.

41. Patel RB, Vaduganathan M, Rikhi A, et al. History of Atrial Fibrillation and Trajectory of Decongestion in Acute Heart Failure. JACC Heart Fail 2019;7(1): 47–55.

42. Roy D, Talajic M, Nattel S, et al. Rhythm control versus rate control for atrial fibrillation and heart failure. N Engl J Med 2008;358(25):2667–77.

43. Moller M, Torp-Pedersen CT, Kober L. Dofetilide in patients with congestive heart failure and left ventricular dysfunction: safety aspects and effect on atrial fibrillation. The Danish Investigators of Arrhythmia and Mortality on Dofetilide (DIAMOND) Study Group. Congest Heart Fail 2001;7(3): 146–50.

44. Ganesan AN, Nandal S, Luker J, et al. Catheter ablation of atrial fibrillation in patients with concomitant left ventricular impairment: a systematic review of efficacy and effect on ejection fraction. Heart Lung Circ 2015;24(3):270–80.

45. Hunter RJ, Berriman TJ, Diab I, et al. A randomized controlled trial of catheter ablation versus medical treatment of atrial fibrillation in heart failure (the CAMTAF trial). Circ Arrhythmia Electrophysiol 2014;7(1):31–8.

46. Jones DG, Haldar SK, Hussain W, et al. A randomized trial to assess catheter ablation versus rate control in the management of persistent atrial fibrillation in heart failure. J Am Coll Cardiol 2013;61(18):1894–903.

47. Verma A, Kalman JM, Callans DJ. Treatment of patients with atrial fibrillation and heart failure with reduced ejection fraction. Circulation 2017; 135(16):1547–63.

48. Prabhu S, Taylor AJ, Costello BT, et al. Catheter Ablation Versus Medical Rate Control in Atrial Fibrillation and Systolic Dysfunction. The CAMERA-MRI Study. J Am Coll Cardiol 2017;70(16):1949–61.

49. Di Biase L, Mohanty P, Mohanty S, et al. Ablation Versus Amiodarone for Treatment of Persistent Atrial Fibrillation in Patients With Congestive Heart Failure and an Implanted Device: Results From the AATAC Multicenter Randomized Trial. Circulation 2016;133(17):1637–44.

50. Marrouche NF, Brachmann J, Andresen D, et al. Catheter Ablation for Atrial Fibrillation with Heart Failure. N Engl J Med 2018;378(5):417–27.

51. January CT, Wann LS, Calkins H, et al. 2019 AHA/ACC/HRS Focused Update of the 2014 AHA/ACC/HRS Guideline for the Management of Patients With Atrial Fibrillation: A Report of the American College of Cardiology/American Heart Association Task Force on Clinical Practice Guidelines and the Heart Rhythm Society in Collaboration With

the Society of Thoracic Surgeons. Circulation 2019; 140(2):e125–51.

52. Goyal P, Almarzooq ZI, Cheung J, et al. Atrial fibrillation and heart failure with preserved ejection fraction: Insights on a unique clinical phenotype from a nationally-representative United States cohort. Int J Cardiol 2018;266:112–8.

53. Zafrir B, Lund LH, Laroche C, et al. Prognostic implications of atrial fibrillation in heart failure with reduced, mid-range, and preserved ejection fraction: a report from 14 964 patients in the European Society of Cardiology Heart Failure Long-Term Registry. Eur Heart J 2018;39(48):4277–84.

54. Abed HS, Wittert GA, Leong DP, et al. Effect of weight reduction and cardiometabolic risk factor management on symptom burden and severity in patients with atrial fibrillation: a randomized clinical trial. JAMA 2013;310(19):2050–60.

55. Lam CSP, Rienstra M, Tay WT, et al. Atrial fibrillation in heart failure with preserved ejection fraction. association with exercise capacity, left ventricular filling pressures, natriuretic peptides, and left atrial volume. JACC Heart Fail 2017;5(2):92–8.

56. Pathak RK, Middeldorp ME, Lau DH, et al. Aggressive risk factor reduction study for atrial fibrillation and implications for the outcome of ablation: the ARREST-AF cohort study. J Am Coll Cardiol 2014; 64(21):2222–31.

57. Kotecha D, Lam CS, Van Veldhuisen DJ, et al. Heart failure with preserved ejection fraction and atrial fibrillation: vicious twins. J Am Coll Cardiol 2016;68(20):2217–28.

58. Cha YM, Wokhlu A, Asirvatham SJ, et al. Success of ablation for atrial fibrillation in isolated left ventricular diastolic dysfunction: a comparison to systolic dysfunction and normal ventricular function. Circ Arrhythmia Electrophysiol 2011;4(5): 724–32.

59. Kelly JP, DeVore AD, Wu J, et al. Rhythm control versus rate control in patients with atrial fibrillation and heart failure with preserved ejection fraction: insights from get with the guidelines-heart failure. J Am Heart Assoc 2019;8(24):e011560.

60. Sobue Y, Watanabe E, Lip GYH, et al. Thromboembolisms in atrial fibrillation and heart failure patients with a preserved ejection fraction (HFpEF) compared to those with a reduced ejection fraction (HFrEF). Heart Vessels 2018;33(4):403–12.

61. Xiong Q, Lau YC, Senoo K, et al. Non-vitamin K antagonist oral anticoagulants (NOACs) in patients with concomitant atrial fibrillation and heart failure: a systemic review and meta-analysis of randomized trials. Eur J Heart Fail 2015;17(11):1192–200.

62. Savarese G, Giugliano RP, Rosano GM, et al. Efficacy and safety of novel oral anticoagulants in patients with atrial fibrillation and heart failure: a meta-analysis. JACC Heart Fail 2016;4(11):870–80.

63. Packer DL, Mark DB, Robb RA, et al. Effect of catheter ablation vs antiarrhythmic drug therapy on mortality, stroke, bleeding, and cardiac arrest among patients with atrial fibrillation: the CABANA randomized clinical trial. JAMA 2019;321(13): 1261–74.

64. Khan MN, Jaïs P, Cummings J, et al. Pulmonary-Vein Isolation for Atrial Fibrillation in Patients with Heart Failure. N Engl J Med 2008;359(17):1778–85.

65. Roglic G. WHO Global report on diabetes: A summary. Int J Noncommun Dis 2016;1(1):3.

66. Control CfD, Prevention. National diabetes statistics report, 2017. Atlanta (GA): Centers for Disease Control and Prevention, US Department of Health and Human Services; 2017.

67. Rowley WR, Bezold C, Arikan Y, et al. Diabetes 2030: Insights from Yesterday, Today, and Future Trends. Popul Health Manag 2017;20(1):6–12.

68. Nichols GA, Gullion CM, Koro CE, et al. The incidence of congestive heart failure in type 2 diabetes: an update. Diabetes care 2004;27(8): 1879–84.

69. Dei Cas A, Fonarow GC, Gheorghiade M, et al. Concomitant Diabetes Mellitus and Heart Failure. Curr Probl Cardiol 2015;40(1):7–43.

70. Dunlay SM, Givertz MM, Aguilar D, et al. Type 2 diabetes mellitus and heart failure, a scientific statement from the American Heart Association and Heart Failure Society of America. J Card Fail 2019;25(8):584–619.

71. Sandesara PB, O'Neal WT, Kelli HM, et al. The prognostic significance of diabetes and microvascular complications in patients with heart failure with preserved ejection fraction. Diabetes Care 2018;41(1):150–5.

72. Kannel WB, McGee DL. Diabetes and cardiovascular disease: the Framingham study. JAMA 1979;241(19):2035–8.

73. Marwick TH, Ritchie R, Shaw JE, et al. Implications of underlying mechanisms for the recognition and management of diabetic cardiomyopathy. J Am Coll Cardiol 2018;71(3):339–51.

74. Dauriz M, Targher G, Laroche C, et al. Association between diabetes and 1-year adverse clinical outcomes in a multinational cohort of ambulatory patients with chronic heart failure: results from the ESC-HFA heart failure long-term registry. Diabetes Care 2017;40(5):671–8.

75. From AM, Leibson CL, Bursi F, et al. Diabetes in heart failure: prevalence and impact on outcome in the population. Am J Med 2006;119(7):591–9.

76. Allen LA, Magid DJ, Gurwitz JH, et al. Risk factors for adverse outcomes by left ventricular ejection fraction in a contemporary heart failure population. Circ Heart Fail 2013;6(4):635–46.

77. McMurray JJV, Solomon SD, Inzucchi SE, et al. Dapagliflozin in patients with heart failure and

reduced ejection fraction. N Engl J Med 2019; 381(21):1995–2008.

78. Das SR, Everett BM, Birtcher KK, et al. 2018 ACC expert consensus decision pathway on novel therapies for cardiovascular risk reduction in patients with type 2 diabetes and atherosclerotic cardiovascular disease: a report of the American College of Cardiology Task Force on Expert Consensus Decision Pathways. J Am Coll Cardiol 2018;72(24): 3200–23.

79. American Diabetes Association. 10. Cardiovascular disease and risk management: Standards of Medical Care in Diabetes—2019. Diabetes Care 2019;42(Supplement 1):S103–23.

80. Castagno D, Baird-Gunning J, Jhund PS, et al. Intensive glycemic control has no impact on the risk of heart failure in type 2 diabetic patients: evidence from a 37,229 patient meta-analysis. Am Heart J 2011;162(5):938–48.e2.

81. Elder DH, Singh JS, Levin D, et al. Mean HbA1c and mortality in diabetic individuals with heart failure: a population cohort study. Eur J Heart Fail 2016;18(1):94–102.

82. Aguilar D, Bozkurt B, Ramasubbu K, et al. Relationship of hemoglobin A1C and mortality in heart failure patients with diabetes. J Am Coll Cardiol 2009; 54(5):422–8.

83. Vaduganathan M, Patel RB, Singh A, et al. Prescription of glucagon-like peptide-1 receptor agonists by cardiologists. J Am Coll Cardiol 2019; 73(12):1596–8.

84. Vaduganathan M, Sathiyakumar V, Singh A, et al. Prescriber Patterns of SGLT2i After Expansions of U.S. Food and Drug Administration Labeling. J Am Coll Cardiol 2018;72(25):3370–2.

85. Patel RB, Al Rifai M, McEvoy JW, et al. Implications of specialist density for diabetes care in the United States. JAMA Cardiol 2019;4(11):1174–5.

86. Gunawan F, Partridge C, Kosiborod M, et al. SUN-149 cardiologist vs. endocrinologist encounters in patients with T2D and CVD: potential implications for glucose-lowering therapy use and education. J Endocr Soc 2019;3(Suppl 1). SUN-149.

87. Davis BR, Piller LB, Cutler JA, et al. Role of diuretics in the prevention of heart failure: the antihypertensive and lipid-lowering treatment to prevent heart attack trial. Circulation 2006;113(18): 2201–10.

88. Bozkurt B, Aguilar D, Deswal A, et al. Contributory risk and management of comorbidities of hypertension, obesity, diabetes mellitus, hyperlipidemia, and metabolic syndrome in chronic heart failure: a scientific statement from the American Heart Association. Circulation 2016;134(23):e535–78.

89. Berl T, Hunsicker LG, Lewis JB, et al. Cardiovascular outcomes in the Irbesartan Diabetic Nephropathy Trial of patients with type 2 diabetes and overt nephropathy. Ann Intern Med 2003; 138(7):542–9.

90. Kasai T, Bradley TD. Obstructive sleep apnea and heart failure: pathophysiologic and therapeutic implications. J Am Coll Cardiol 2011;57(2):119–27.

91. Komajda M, Anker SD, Cowie MR, et al. Physicians' adherence to guideline-recommended medications in heart failure with reduced ejection fraction: data from the QUALIFY global survey. Eur J Heart Fail 2016;18(5):514–22.

92. Peri-Okonny PA, Mi X, Khariton Y, et al. Target doses of heart failure medical therapy and blood pressure: insights from the CHAMP-HF Registry. JACC Heart Fail 2019;7(4):350–8.

93. Malha L, Mann SJ. Loop diuretics in the treatment of hypertension. Curr Hypertens Rep 2016;18(4): 27.

94. Colucci WS, Kolias TJ, Adams KF, et al. Metoprolol reverses left ventricular remodeling in patients with asymptomatic systolic dysfunction: the REversal of VEntricular Remodeling with Toprol-XL (REVERT) trial. Circulation 2007;116(1):49–56.

95. Exner DV, Dries DL, Waclawiw MA, et al. Beta-adrenergic blocking agent use and mortality in patients with asymptomatic and symptomatic left ventricular systolic dysfunction: a post hoc analysis of the studies of left ventricular dysfunction. J Am Coll Cardiol 1999;33(4):916–23.

96. SOLVD Investigators, Yusuf S, Pitt B, Davis CE, et al. Effect of enalapril on mortality and the development of heart failure in asymptomatic patients with reduced left ventricular ejection fractions. N Engl J Med 1992;327(10):685–91.

97. Jong P, Yusuf S, Rousseau MF, et al. Effect of enalapril on 12-year survival and life expectancy in patients with left ventricular systolic dysfunction: a follow-up study. Lancet 2003;361(9372):1843–8.

98. Ekeruo IA, Solhpour A, Taegtmeyer H. Metformin in diabetic patients with heart failure: safe and effective? Curr Cardiovasc Risk Rep 2013;7(6):417–22.

99. Rosenstock J, Kahn SE, Johansen OE, et al. Effect of linagliptin vs glimepiride on major adverse cardiovascular outcomes in patients with type 2 diabetes: the CAROLINA randomized clinical trial. JAMA 2019;322(12):1155–66.

100. Group NS, Holman RR, Haffner SM, et al. Effect of nateglinide on the incidence of diabetes and cardiovascular events. N Engl J Med 2010;362(16): 1463–76.

101. Holman RR, Coleman RL, Chan JCN, et al. Effects of acarbose on cardiovascular and diabetes outcomes in patients with coronary heart disease and impaired glucose tolerance (ACE): a randomised, double-blind, placebo-controlled trial. Lancet Diabetes Endocrinol 2017;5(11):877–86.

102. Basal insulin and cardiovascular and other outcomes in dysglycemia. N Engl J Med 2012; 367(4):319–28.

103. Dormandy JA, Charbonnel B, Eckland DJ, et al. Secondary prevention of macrovascular events in patients with type 2 diabetes in the PROactive Study (PROspective pioglitAzone Clinical Trial In macroVascular Events): a randomised controlled trial. Lancet 2005;366(9493):1279–89.

104. Home PD, Pocock SJ, Beck-Nielsen H, et al. Rosiglitazone evaluated for cardiovascular outcomes in oral agent combination therapy for type 2 diabetes (RECORD): a multicentre, randomised, open-label trial. Lancet 2009;373(9681):2125–35.

105. Pfeffer MA, Claggett B, Diaz R, et al. Lixisenatide in patients with type 2 diabetes and acute coronary syndrome. N Engl J Med 2015;373(23):2247–57.

106. Marso SP, Daniels GH, Brown-Frandsen K, et al. Liraglutide and cardiovascular outcomes in type 2 diabetes. N Engl J Med 2016;375(4):311–22.

107. Marso SP, Bain SC, Consoli A, et al. Semaglutide and cardiovascular outcomes in patients with type 2 diabetes. N Engl J Med 2016;375(19): 1834–44.

108. Holman RR, Bethel MA, Mentz RJ, et al. Effects of once-weekly exenatide on cardiovascular outcomes in type 2 diabetes. N Engl J Med 2017; 377(13):1228–39.

109. Hernandez AF, Green JB, Janmohamed S, et al. Albiglutide and cardiovascular outcomes in patients with type 2 diabetes and cardiovascular disease (Harmony Outcomes): a double-blind, randomised placebo-controlled trial. Lancet 2018;392(10157): 1519–29.

110. Scirica BM, Bhatt DL, Braunwald E, et al. Saxagliptin and cardiovascular outcomes in patients with type 2 diabetes mellitus. N Engl J Med 2013; 369(14):1317–26.

111. White WB, Cannon CP, Heller SR, et al. Alogliptin after acute coronary syndrome in patients with type 2 diabetes. N Engl J Med 2013;369(14): 1327–35.

112. Zannad F, Cannon CP, Cushman WC, et al. Heart failure and mortality outcomes in patients with type 2 diabetes taking alogliptin versus placebo in EXAMINE: a multicentre, randomised, double-blind trial. Lancet 2015;385(9982):2067–76.

113. Green JB, Bethel MA, Armstrong PW, et al. Effect of sitagliptin on cardiovascular outcomes in type 2 diabetes. N Engl J Med 2015;373(3):232–42.

114. Fitchett D, Butler J, van de Borne P, et al. Effects of empagliflozin on risk for cardiovascular death and heart failure hospitalization across the spectrum of heart failure risk in the EMPA-REG OUTCOME® trial. Eur Heart J 2017;39(5):363–70.

115. Neal B, Perkovic V, Mahaffey KW, et al. Canagliflozin and cardiovascular and renal events in type 2 diabetes. N Engl J Med 2017;377(7):644–57.

116. Wiviott SD, Raz I, Bonaca MP, et al. Dapagliflozin and cardiovascular outcomes in type 2 diabetes. N Engl J Med 2019;380(4):347–57.

Systematizing Heart Failure Population Health

Prateeti Khazanie, MD, MPH*, Larry A. Allen, MD, MHS

KEYWORDS

- Heart failure • Population health • Population medicine • Health policy • Process improvement
- Value

KEY POINTS

- Population health and population health management/medicine are highly relevant to delivering high-value, patient-centered care for patients with heart failure.
- There are opportunities to systematize processes of care for the different American College of Cardiology/American Heart Association heart failure stages.
- Future efforts to optimize population health management/medicine will require integration of complex data and multidisciplinary collaboration.

INTRODUCTION

The United States spends more money on health care per capita compared with other high-income countries, yet has lower life expectancy and worse health outcomes.[1] The reasons for this higher spending are thought to be driven by higher prices and greater utilization of medical technology rather than routine clinic visits and social services.[1] Heart failure affects more than 6 million people in the United States with a total annual cost of more than $30.7 billion,[2] making heart failure one of the most common, expensive, and resource intensive chronic conditions in health care.

Future solutions to help curb spending include shifts in payment models to reward health care providers based on their patient population's health outcomes.

Population health is an approach to health care that aims to improve the health of a population. It is defined as "the health outcomes of a group of individuals, including the distribution of such outcomes within the group."[3] Population health sometimes gets confused with public health, but they are different. Public health is what "we as a society do collectively to assure the conditions in which people can be healthy"[4] and involves government health policies. Population health integrates nonclinical determinants of health with measures of health and health care, monitoring and reporting factors that may influence an individual's health outcomes (**Fig. 1**).

Policymakers estimate that 80% of what affects health outcomes is associated with factors outside the health care system, such as health behaviors, environment, psychosocial and economic factors, and others.[5] Because of the large number of factors at play, population health policies have to focus on economic tradeoffs in health care because resources are always limited, and systems must determine the cost-effectiveness of resource allocation to initiatives targeting multiple determinants of health.[6] In other words, health systems must provide high-value care, defined by "patient outcomes achieved relative to the cost of care required to achieve those patient outcomes," while also focusing on the health of the overall population (**Fig. 2**).[7]

Division of Cardiology, University of Colorado School of Medicine, 12631 East 17th Avenue, Mail Stop B130, Aurora, CO 80045, USA
* Corresponding author. Division of Cardiology, University of Colorado School of Medicine, 12631 East 17th Avenue, Mail Stop B130, Aurora, CO 80045.
E-mail address: prateeti.khazanie@cuanschutz.edu

Heart Failure Clin 16 (2020) 457–466
https://doi.org/10.1016/j.hfc.2020.06.006
1551-7136/20/© 2020 Elsevier Inc. All rights reserved.

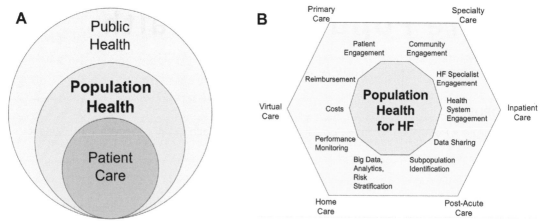

Fig. 1. Population health in heart failure (HF). (*A*) Population health is "the health outcomes of a group of individuals, including the distribution of such outcomes within the group."[3] Population health expands on traditional patient care by including factors such as health behaviors, environment, psychosocial and economic factors, and others. Public health is what society collectively does to improve health with the involvement of government policies, and population health help fills in gaps in public health initiatives and focuses on health outcomes. (*B*) Population health management/medicine is the "process of strategically and proactively managing clinical and financial opportunities to improve health outcomes and patient engagement, while also reducing costs."[6] Population health in heart failure coordinates primary, specialty, inpatient, postacute, home, and virtual care to improve health outcomes.

Population health is 1 of the 3 pillars of the Institute for Healthcare Improvement's Triple Aim.[8] The Triple Aim is the simultaneous pursuit of 3 linked goals—improving the individual experience of care, reducing per capita cost of care, and optimizing the health of populations; the Quadruple Aim adds the well-being of the health care team, a component that is particularly important in heart

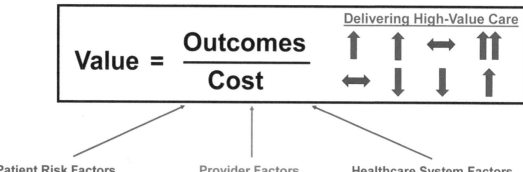

Fig. 2. The value equation. Health care value is defined as patient outcomes achieved relative to the cost of care required to achieve those patient outcomes.[7] Patient, provider, and health care system factors all contribute to health care value. Delivery of high-value care occurs in different scenarios, including (1) positive outcomes with net even costs, (2) positive outcomes with low costs, (3) equivocal outcomes but low cost, and (4) very positive outcomes at high cost. In the end, the lens from which value is judged is important, and it is different for patients, providers, payers, and health systems.

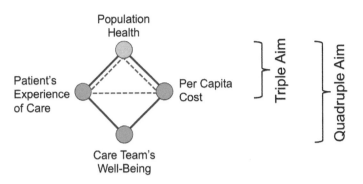

Fig. 3. The Triple and Quadruple Aims. Population health is a major goal of both the Triple and Quadruple Aims. The Triple Aim includes 3 goals: (1) optimizing population health, (2) improving the individual patient's experience of care, and (3) reducing per capita cost of care. The Quadruple Aim adds a fourth goal: the well-being of the health care team.

failure due to intense and sometimes burdensome chronic care management (**Fig. 3**).[8,9] These constructs have drawn extra attention to the necessity of thinking beyond the individual patient and also to the health of populations. Rapid changes in the past decade in health care reimbursements, health policies, and provider incentives have shifted previously siloed, fee-for-service payment structures to reimbursing for high-quality health care for specific populations, also known as population health management or population medicine. The goals of population health are to improve health outcomes and quality, to proactively address factors affecting at-risk patients, to identify optimal disease management programs, to improve care delivery by leveraging technology and data so providers can improve care coordination, and to create cost-effective health systems that reduce financial burden on patients and providers. These aspirational goals of population health and population health management/medicine are particularly evocative for chronic diseases such as heart failure.

HEART FAILURE POPULATION HEALTH MANAGEMENT

Health systems are now attempting to transition from reactive to proactive structures for complex disease management. In traditional health care systems, health care teams are reactive, patients must bring problems to the attention of their teams, and the number of heart failure patients in the systems are unknown. In contrast, systems that focus on population health have health care teams identify all patients in the system with heart failure, risk stratify the population into different groups based on stage of disease and relevant care pathways, and then contact patients who may benefit from proactive changes to care; the denominator of patients with heart failure is known and their data are collected in registries. In order to achieve population health in heart failure, health

systems and clinicians need to measure, monitor, and identify trends in patients' health in order to address process improvement.

Fortunately, there are many guideline-directed medical therapies, device therapies, and processes of care that have been proved to improve outcomes for patients with heart failure with reduced ejection fraction, and there is hope for future therapies for heart failure with preserved ejection fraction.[10] However, heart failure clinics and specialists can only see a minority of all patients with heart failure, and when they do they may not have the time and processes in place to ensure appropriate consideration of all high-value care options. Thus, in order to fulfill the Quadruple Aim—to provide individualized, cost-effective care that improves the health of heart failure populations and also maintains health care providers' well-being—it is imperative that health care systems focus on population health management systems. Such systems focus on the "process of strategically and proactively managing clinical and financial opportunities to improve health outcomes and patient engagement, while also reducing costs."[6] The purpose of population health management/medicine in heart failure is to use patient health information aggregated from health information technology systems to understand how different heart failure populations are treated and then to understand their outcomes based on these treatments. It also identifies optimal treatment programs and at-risk patients to enable early intervention.

Concomitant with a focus on population health and population health management, health systems must provide high-value care. However, value is extremely difficult to define because the lens for judging outcomes is different based on whether one is looking at it from the health system finance perspective, payer perspective, provider perspective, or patient perspective. One of the more widely accepted definitions of value as proposed by Porter[11] states that health outcomes should reflect the "health circumstances most relevant to patients," but regardless, perspective is important, and providers should get paid to "do the right thing." Thus, contemporary shifts in health care delivery systems from fee-for-service to value-based payment models create potential opportunities to address population health in chronic disease processes, such as heart failure.

SYSTEMATIZING PROCESSES OF HEART FAILURE CARE BASED ON DISEASE SEVERITY

There are significant opportunities to systematize processes of heart failure care. Many prior interventions have focused on treating diseases that can lead to heart failure, and the incidence of new-onset heart failure is decreasing.[12] However, once patients develop chronic heart failure, providers and health systems do a poor job of proactively managing their disease with guideline-directed medical therapy intensification and disease management. Rather, once patients have heart failure, the approach has been more reactive, and thus, health systems and payers use copious resources in hospitalizations and preventing readmissions rather than preventing the first hospitalization. In the future, the approaches to tackling population health management will need to be different based on patients' American College of Cardiology/American Heart Association heart failure stage, ranging from pre-vention to end-of-life. Depending on the stage of disease, health systems and organizations will need to design, deliver, coordinate, and pay for high-quality health services to manage the Quadruple Aim for a population using the optimal resources available.

American College of Cardiology/American Heart Association Stage A

Perhaps the greatest role for population health to improve heart failure is by preventing incident disease. In the future, population health data mining must include early identification of patients who are at high risk for heart failure before they ever present with left ventricular dysfunction or symptomatic disease. Many traditional and existing population health–focused interventions have been designed to address diseases that are risk factors for heart failure, such as smoking cessation, treatments for high blood pressure (medication, low-sodium diet, active lifestyle), treatment of high cholesterol, regular exercise, and other preventative interventions.[13–16] Optimizing such upstream interventions and creatively deploying them in populations, particularly high-risk

populations, will help reduce progression to future disease expression.

American College of Cardiology/American Heart Association Stage B

For patients with pre-heart failure who have systolic left ventricular dysfunction but no active symptoms, early identification and treatment is essential. This population is at considerable risk for development of symptomatic heart failure (Stages C and D). Because of the increasing ability to identify low left ventricular ejection fraction with field coding (see Byrd and colleagues' article, "Defragmenting Heart Failure Care: Medical Records Integration," in this issue), left ventricular hypertrophy on routine electrocardiograms, and increasing availability of natriuretic peptides and other biomarkers, this should be a key future target for population health interventions triggered by improvements in data science.

Data from randomized controlled trials have established neurohormonal antagonist medications—beta-blockers, angiotensin-converting enzyme inhibitors, angiotensin receptor blockers, angiotensin receptor-neprilysin inhibitors, and aldosterone antagonists—as the foundation of therapy for patients with systolic left ventricular dysfunction. Use of these medications is recommended by multiple clinical practice guidelines[17,18] and is critical to improving outcomes for patients with systolic dysfunction. Unfortunately, medication adherence and intensification has not been thoroughly studied in this population, which makes it ripe for future investigation.

American College of Cardiology/American Heart Association Stage C

Once patients have symptomatic heart failure, many interventions have been tested, but their uptake and effectiveness in real-world settings has been limited. Personnel-based interventions (eg, disease management programs, transition coaches) have been popular but can be resource intensive and often require trained personnel. Diuretic-based interventions to control fluid status (eg, furosemide dosing based on daily weights) are the default therapeutic strategy for patients following HF hospitalization. However, focusing on diuretic titration is not evidence based,[19] and patients are frequently still congested after a hospitalization for acute heart failure.[20,21]

More than 80% of current costs and resources are currently spent in treating prevalent disease (stage C heart failure) largely due to fragmented care.[2] Although there have been multiple randomized clinical trials showing clinical efficacy of guideline-directed medical therapies for heart failure, data show that therapeutic inertia is widespread with underuse of guideline-directed medical therapies for heart failure and slow uptake of new therapies.[22,23] Unfortunately, longitudinal gaps in pharmacotherapy are present, and the magnitude and causes of specific gaps in intensification, monitoring, and adherence for heart failure therapies remain poorly defined. Moreover, the patient and provider factors that contribute to suboptimal pharmacotherapy are largely unknown. Prior inpatient and outpatient quality initiatives (eg, OPTIMIZE-HF,[24] GWTG-HF,[25,26] IMPROVE-HF,[27] PINNACLE,[28] and CHAMP-HF[22,29]) have focused on initiation of heart failure therapies and longitudinal use of these therapies in the care continuum. Appropriate intensification, safety monitoring, and adherence are all necessary for these therapies to effectively reduce readmissions. If prior initiatives such as these are combined with other data, their effect on population health medicine could be substantial. Finally, complex medication regimens and polypharmacy make medication nonadherence a real obstacle in heart failure management.[30,31] In order to improve medication adherence, studies can monitor fills and actively engage patients in their own care. Future interventions will require creative solutions with patient engagement, caregiver and community activation, disease management programs, and multipronged approaches to improve outcomes.

American College of Cardiology/American Heart Association Stage D

By the time patients develop more end-stage, advanced heart failure with symptoms refractory to traditional medical and device therapies, patients often benefit from appropriate referral for advanced heart failure and palliative care. Advanced heart failure therapies, such as heart transplantation and mechanical circulatory support, require careful patient selection and are not for everyone.[32–35] These therapies are associated with the potential for high rewards and also for high risks. For health care systems focusing on population health, the highest risk patients may not always return the most clinical improvement or best outcomes, and, thus, long-term investments may be more high value in patients with moderate or rising risk rather than end-stage disease. Currently, there are considerable variations and health disparities in the types of patients who receive advanced heart failure therapies,[36,37] and referrals to hospice are often too late.[38,39] The relatively unpredictable course of stage D heart failure makes timing of referrals for higher levels of care and hospice very challenging, particularly across populations. Patient preferences are varied, advanced care directives are difficult to systematize, and patients' values can change over time. Future efforts to improve population health for patients with end-stage heart failure will require careful and timely patient referral, evaluation, and selection for heart transplantation, mechanical support, or hospice.

PAYMENT POLICY CHANGES TO PROMOTE POPULATION HEALTH

In response to the need to improve the patient experience and quality of care and to curb rising health care costs, the health care industry is gradually shifting from fee-for-service reimbursement to value-based models. One of the early examples of this shift in the heart failure world is the Hospital Readmissions Reduction Program (HRRP). After the Medicare Payment Advisory Commission first advised Congress that readmissions may be a target to reduce costs and improve patient care in 2007,[40] the Centers for Medicare and Medicaid Services (CMS) started publicly reporting 30-day hospital risk-standardized readmission rates after hospital discharge as an indicator of quality and efficiency of care on its Hospital Compare Website in 2009.[41,42] After this, the mandatory pay-for-performance HRRP was created under the 2010 Patient Protection and Affordable Care Act with readmissions reporting beginning in 2010 and the penalty phase beginning in 2012.[43] This public reporting was designed to reduce costs, break down silos of care, and improve care transitions and communication with outside providers. Although the HRRP was aimed at multiple diagnoses, heart failure has been the main driver of the HRRP penalties.

The Veterans' Administration (VA), the largest integrated health care system in the United States, has low rates of readmission,[44] but data suggest that the readmission metric may not be as useful in the VA system because it does not have the clinical volume to pick up differences between different VA hospitals.[45] To be included in CMS reporting, hospitals have to have at least 25 heart failure admissions annually, and 38% of VA hospitals did not meet this volume requirement for heart failure readmissions.[45] CMS 30-day risk-standardized readmission rates may not be a useful measure to distinguish performance between different VA hospitals, given low hospital-level volume for these readmissions. Thus, readmissions are an imperfect outcome measure for the VA and many smaller hospitals but are a first step in the transition from fee-for-service to value-based payments.

Accountable Care Organizations (ACOs) are becoming one of the most common approaches to addressing federal incentive and penalty programs such as value-based purchasing. ACOs are groups of doctors, hospitals, and other health care providers, who come together voluntarily to give coordinated high-quality care to the Medicare patients they serve. Coordinated care helps ensure that patients, especially the chronically ill, get the right care at the right time, with the goal of avoiding unnecessary duplication of services and preventing medical errors. When an ACO succeeds in both delivering high-quality care and spending health care dollars more wisely, it will share in the savings it achieves for the Medicare program. Unfortunately, these gains have been modest in pilot programs, and further changes to the system are likely required before significant gains in health care value can be achieved.[46,47] More recently, ACOs have worked to reduce readmissions. Kaiser Permanente showed a reduction in 30-day all-cause readmission rates with transitional care programs and bundling elements.[48] Another example is the Accountable Care Collaborative in Colorado that focused on Medicaid payment and delivery reforms and showed 8.6% fewer hospital readmissions than nonparticipating enrollees in the first year.[49]

CHALLENGES AND EVOLUTION
Cohort Definition

One of the major challenges in population health for heart failure is appropriate cohort definition and prioritization of interventions. Currently, most health care systems use administrative codes (eg, ICD-10 and CPT codes) to define heart failure cohorts. Solely relying on these codes will miss patients who should have been included in the cohort and who could have benefited from population health interventions. Identification of cohorts will be more effective if there is integration of supplemental administrative codes (eg, ICD-10 codes for volume overload or risk of hemodynamic instability), medications (eg, patients taking aggressive doses of diuretics for volume management), imaging studies and laboratory tests (eg, ejection fraction and biomarkers such as brain natriuretic peptide), along with other data. Distinguishing patients with heart failure with reduced versus preserved ejection fraction will be imperative because the ideal processes of care for heart failure with preserved ejection fraction are less clear. Finally, identifying patients in the cohort who can

be managed by the appropriate provider (eg, primary care provider, cardiology, or advanced heart failure specialist) will be imperative. Heart failure clinics specializing in disease management can only see a fraction of patients with heart failure.[50] Thus, heart failure specialists and health systems must partner with primary care physicians and community groups on the frontline to provide optimal, high-value care for patients with heart failure.

Challenges with the electronic health records are addressed in detail in Byrd and colleagues' article, "Defragmenting Heart Failure Care: Medical Records Integration," in this issue, but future efforts to optimize population health and population health management/medicine will require widely accessible, structured data sources. Electronic health records are currently designed for a fee-for-service system, focusing on diagnoses and billing. However, in a population health–focused system, there needs to be greater transparency for the cost of care at the point of care.

Patient Engagement

In addition to partnering with primary care physicians and community groups and optimizing data acquisition and tracking, future interventions will need to incorporate patient perspectives into decision-making. A critical gap is the failure to empower patients to engage more directly in their care. Patients have a direct stake in making sure they are getting efficacious treatments, want to be involved in decisions about their treatments, and if engaged are more likely to adhere to them. New studies, such as the Electronic Health Record-leveraged, Patient-centered, Intensification of Chronic Care for Heart Failure (EPIC-HF) trial and the Personalized Patient Data and Behavioral Nudges to Improve Adherence to Chronic Cardiovascular Medications (Nudge) trial, are testing the effectiveness of patient empowerment and activation for optimization of medication plans.[51,52]

In EPIC-HF,[51] patients with heart failure with reduced ejection fraction enrolled in the intervention arm are receiving, by email and/or text, a link to (1) a short patient engagement video around heart failure medications and (2) a link to an online PDF of a medication checklist. Patients enrolled in the control arm do not receive any materials at any point of time and receive their usual care. For both arms, medication changes in patient medical records are being assessed before and after clinic visits to measure the effectiveness of the intervention; surveys are also being compared before and after clinic visits to determine the effectiveness of the intervention. The Nudge trial[52] is a pragmatic patient-level randomized intervention using a mixed methods approach and cell phone technology to facilitate medication adherence for chronic cardiovascular medications. Patients are being identified through pharmacy refill data to have a 7-day gap in prescribed cardiovascular medication refills and are being randomized to 1 of 4 arms—usual care, generic reminder text, optimized nudge text, and optimized nudge plus artificial intelligence chatbot to assess barriers filling the medication. Trials such as these are testing novel interventions and whether patient engagement improves medication adherence and clinical outcomes.

Other methods of patient engagement will include incorporating patient-generated health data and clinical perspectives, including remote monitoring with CardioMEMS, devices, wearables, shared decision-making with multiple decision aids, and incorporation of patient's perspectives on costs of care.[53–56] Patient-centered care has become the forefront of health policy as exemplified by the Centers for Medicare and Medicaid Services requirements for the use of evidence-based decision aids for left atrial appendage closure devices and primary prevention implantable cardioverter defibrillators.[57–59]

Redefining Hospitalization Metrics and Choosing Measurable Outcomes

As we evolve to move from silos of care to more patient-centered care, it will be important to recognize that, although imperfect, programs such as the HRRP are a first step in curbing spending and improving value-based care. The readmission measure is very hospital-centric, and it would be better to avoid hospitalization in the first place rather than focusing solely on readmission. To improve the readmission measure, policies could include total hospitalizations, all postdischarge care (including observation stations and emergency department visits), healthy days at home, potentially preventable admission for inpatient hospital care, potentially preventable emergency department visit, and mortality rates after inpatient hospital stay.[60,61] Health systems need to focus beyond hospital walls and incorporate and target psycho-socioeconomic issues to reduce disease disparities and inequities. Physicians will need to codesign pragmatic interventions and processes that use their health care teams—nurses, dieticians, pharmacists, nutritionists, health coaches—and collaborate with community organizations.

DATA INTEGRATION TO ACHIEVE HIGH-VALUE CARE IN POPULATION HEALTH

Patients with heart failure generate large amounts of complex data with multiple clinical encounters and diagnostic tests. Their data are frequently disconnected and siloed because patients are seen by different providers and health systems and get clinical tests from different companies and laboratory systems. Current information technology systems are not designed to capture these different data and link them to financial reimbursement data.

Moving forward, in order to optimally integrate population health data for heart failure, accomplish the Quadruple Aim, and achieve high-value care for patients, health systems will need to combine several major categories of data—clinical information from the patient electronic health records, diagnostics and genomic data from laboratories, financial data from billing groups, social determinants of health data, patient and caregiver satisfaction information, and provider well-being data. Thus, payers will need to partner more with health systems and policymakers in collecting and integrating clinical, diagnostic, and financial information in the future. Database creation will require more granular diagnosis codes and ejection fraction to help define the population and may require tools such as natural language processing.[62] It will also require linking medication, laboratory, clinical encounter, and device data to identify patients who are being potentially under- and over-treated. After patients are identified, health systems will need to prioritize interventions balancing risk and costs.

SUMMARY

Optimal population health and population health management of patients with heart failure requires a shift in our treatment paradigm from reactive treatment to proactive prevention. Such prevention includes primary prevention to reduced incident disease and secondary prevention of heart failure exacerbations, hospitalizations, guideline-directed medical therapy optimization, standardization of advanced heart failure therapies, and smoother transitions to end-of-life care. This can only be done through systems that break down silos of care and think about care provision longitudinally from the patient perspective. Heart failure clinicians share a collective responsibility to expand on prior quality initiatives and to collaborate with health systems and patients in order to move from fee-for-service to population-based approaches that emphasize the provision of high-value care in the community and improve outcomes for patients living with heart failure.

DISCLOSURE

Dr P. Khazanie has nothing to disclose. Dr L.A. Allen has received consulting fees from ACI Clinical, Amgen, Boston Scientific, Cytokinetics, and Novartis.

Funding: Dr P. Khazanie has institutional research grant support from National Institutes of Health (K23 HL145122) and the Center for Women's Health Research, University of Colorado Anschutz Medical Campus. Dr L.A. Allen has received grant funding from the American Heart Association, the National Institutes of Health, and the Patient Centered Outcomes Research Institute.

REFERENCES

1. The Commonwealth Fund. U.S. Health Care from a Global Perspective. Available at: https://www.commonwealthfund.org/publications/issue-briefs/2015/oct/us-health-care-global-perspective?redirect_source=/publications/issue-briefs/2015/oct/us-health-care-from-a-global-perspective. Accessed January 11, 2020.

2. Benjamin EJ, Muntner P, Alonso A, et al. Heart disease and stroke statistics-2019 update: a report from the American Heart Association. Circulation 2019;139(10):e56–528.

3. Kindig D, Stoddart G. What is population health? Am J Public Health 2003;93(3):380–3.

4. Institute of Medicine (US) Committee for the Study of the Future of Public Health. The future of public health. Washington, DC: National Academies Press (US); 1988. Available at: https://www.ncbi.nlm.nih.gov/books/NBK218218/doi: 10.17226/1091. Accessed January 12, 2020.

5. Robert Wood Johnson Foundation. County Health Rankings Key Findings Report. 2015. Available at: https://www.rwjf.org/en/library/research/2015/03/2015-county-health-rankings-key-findings-report.html. Accessed January 11, 2020.

6. What are we talking about when we talk about population health? Health Aff Blog 2015. https://doi.org/10.1377/hblog20150406.046151. Accessed November 11, 2019.

7. Bradley SM, Strauss CE, Ho PM. Value in cardiovascular care. Heart 2017;103(16):1238–43.

8. Institute for Healthcare Improvement. The IHI Triple Aim. Available at: http://www.ihi.org/Engage/Initiatives/TripleAim/Pages/default.aspx. Accessed November 19, 2019.

9. Bodenheimer T, Sinsky C. From triple to quadruple aim: care of the patient requires care of the provider. Ann Fam Med 2014;12(6):573–6.

10. Vaduganathan M, Claggett BL, Desai AS, et al. Prior heart failure hospitalization, clinical outcomes, and response to sacubitril/valsartan compared with valsartan in HFpEF. J Am Coll Cardiol 2019;75(3):245–54.

11. Porter ME. What is value in health care? N Engl J Med 2010;363(26):2477–81.

12. Chen J, Normand SL, Wang Y, et al. National and regional trends in heart failure hospitalization and mortality rates for Medicare beneficiaries, 1998-2008. JAMA 2011;306(15):1669–78.

13. Population Based Smoking Cessation. Proceedings of a Conference on What Works to Influence Cessation in the General Population. Available at: https://cancercontrol.cancer.gov/brp/tcrb/monographs/12/entire_monograph-12.pdf. Accessed January 10, 2020.

14. Victor RG, Lynch K, Li N, et al. A cluster-randomized trial of blood-pressure reduction in black barbershops. N Engl J Med 2018;378(14):1291–301.

15. Aspry KE, Furman R, Karalis DG, et al. Effect of health information technology interventions on lipid management in clinical practice: a systematic review of randomized controlled trials. J Clin Lipidol 2013;7(6):546–60.

16. Lavie CJ, Thomas RJ, Squires RW, et al. Exercise training and cardiac rehabilitation in primary and secondary prevention of coronary heart disease. Mayo Clin Proc 2009;84(4):373–83.

17. Yancy CW, Jessup M, Bozkurt B, et al. 2013 ACCF/AHA guideline for the management of heart failure: a report of the American College of Cardiology Foundation/American Heart Association Task Force on practice guidelines. Circulation 2013;128(16):e240–327.

18. Yancy CW, Jessup M, Bozkurt B, et al. 2017 ACC/AHA/HFSA Focused Update of the 2013 ACCF/AHA Guideline for the Management of Heart Failure: A Report of the American College of Cardiology/American Heart Association Task Force on Clinical Practice Guidelines and the Heart Failure Society of America. Circulation 2017;136(6):e137–61.

19. Faris RF, Flather M, Purcell H, et al. Diuretics for heart failure. Cochrane Database Syst Rev 2012;(2):Cd003838.

20. Lala A, McNulty SE, Mentz RJ, et al. Relief and Recurrence of Congestion During and After Hospitalization for Acute Heart Failure: Insights From Diuretic Optimization Strategy Evaluation in Acute Decompensated Heart Failure (DOSE-AHF) and Cardiorenal Rescue Study in Acute Decompensated Heart Failure (CARESS-HF). Circ Heart Fail 2015;8(4):741–8.

21. Fudim M, Hernandez AF, Felker GM. Role of volume redistribution in the congestion of heart failure. J Am Heart Assoc 2017;6(8):e006817.

22. Greene SJ, Fonarow GC, DeVore AD, et al. Titration of medical therapy for heart failure with reduced ejection fraction. J Am Coll Cardiol 2019;73(19):2365–83.

23. Bhagat AA, Greene SJ, Vaduganathan M, et al. Initiation, continuation, switching, and withdrawal of heart failure medical therapies during hospitalization. JACC Heart Fail 2019;7(1):1–12.

24. Fonarow GC, Abraham WT, Albert NM, et al. Organized Program to Initiate Lifesaving Treatment in Hospitalized Patients with Heart Failure (OPTIMIZE-HF): rationale and design. Am Heart J 2004;148(1):43–51.

25. Krantz MJ, Ambardekar AV, Kaltenbach L, et al. Patterns and predictors of evidence-based medication continuation among hospitalized heart failure patients (from Get With the Guidelines-Heart Failure). Am J Cardiol 2011;107(12):1818–23.

26. Heidenreich PA, Hernandez AF, Yancy CW, et al. Get With The Guidelines program participation, process of care, and outcome for Medicare patients hospitalized with heart failure. Circ Cardiovasc Qual Outcomes 2012;5(1):37–43.

27. Fonarow GC, Albert NM, Curtis AB, et al. Improving evidence-based care for heart failure in outpatient cardiology practices: primary results of the Registry to Improve the Use of Evidence-Based Heart Failure Therapies in the Outpatient Setting (IMPROVE HF). Circulation 2010;122(6):585–96.

28. Peterson PN, Chan PS, Spertus JA, et al. Practice-level variation in use of recommended medications among outpatients with heart failure: Insights from the NCDR PINNACLE program. Circ Heart Fail 2013;6(6):1132–8.

29. Greene SJ, Butler J, Albert NM, et al. Medical therapy for heart failure with reduced ejection fraction: the CHAMP-HF registry. J Am Coll Cardiol 2018;72(4):351–66.

30. Allen LA, Fonarow GC, Liang L, et al. Medication initiation burden required to comply with heart failure guideline recommendations and hospital quality measures. Circulation 2015;132(14):1347–53.

31. Reed BN, Rodgers JE, Sueta CA. Polypharmacy in heart failure: drugs to use and avoid. Heart Fail Clin 2014;10(4):577–90.

32. Khazanie P, Rogers JG. Patient selection for left ventricular assist devices. Congest Heart Fail 2011;17(5):227–34.

33. Fanaroff AC, DeVore AD, Mentz RJ, et al. Patient selection for advanced heart failure therapy referral. Crit Pathw Cardiol 2014;13(1):1–5.

34. Kim JH, Singh R, Pagani FD, et al. Ventricular assist device therapy in older patients with heart failure: characteristics and outcomes. J Card Fail 2016;22(12):981–7.

35. Dunlay SM, Park SJ, Joyce LD, et al. Frailty and outcomes after implantation of left ventricular assist device as destination therapy. J Heart Lung Transplant 2014;33(4):359–65.

36. Khazanie P. REVIVAL of the sex disparities debate: are women denied, never referred, or ineligible for heart replacement therapies? JACC Heart Fail 2019;7(7):612–4.

37. Breathett K, Yee E, Pool N, et al. Does race influence decision making for advanced heart failure therapies? J Am Heart Assoc 2019;8(22):e013592.

38. Warraich HJ, Xu H, DeVore AD, et al. Trends in hospice discharge and relative outcomes among medicare patients in the get with the guidelines-heart failure registry. JAMA Cardiol 2018;3(10):917–26.

39. Cross SH, Warraich HJ. Changes in the place of death in the United States. N Engl J Med 2019;381(24):2369–70.

40. Medicare Payment Advisory Commission. Report to the Congress: Promoting Greater Efficiency in Medicare. 2007. Available at: http://www.medpac.gov/docs/default-source/reports/Jun07_EntireReport.pdf. Accessed December 18, 2020.

41. DeVore AD, Hammill BG, Hardy NC, et al. Has public reporting of hospital readmission rates affected patient outcomes?: analysis of medicare claims data. J Am Coll Cardiol 2016;67(8):963–72.

42. Joynt KE, Orav EJ, Zheng J, et al. Public reporting of mortality rates for hospitalized medicare patients and trends in mortality for reported conditions. Ann Intern Med 2016;165(3):153–60.

43. Centers for Medicare and Medicaid Services. Readmissions Reduction Program (HRRP). Available at: https://www.cms.gov/Medicare/Medicare-Fee-for-Service-Payment/AcuteInpatientPPS/Readmissions-Reduction-Program. Accessed January 7, 2020.

44. Kaboli PJ, Go JT, Hockenberry J, et al. Associations between reduced hospital length of stay and 30-day readmission rate and mortality: 14-year experience in 129 veterans affairs hospitals. Ann Intern Med 2012;157(12):837–45.

45. Wray CM, Vali M, Walter LC, et al. Examining the utility of 30-day readmission rates and hospital profiling in the veterans health administration. J Hosp Med 2019;14(5):266–71.

46. McWilliams JM, Hatfield LA, Chernew ME, et al. Early performance of accountable care organizations in medicare. N Engl J Med 2016;374(24):2357–66.

47. McClellan M, Udayakumar K, Thoumi A, et al. Improving care and lowering costs: evidence and lessons from a global analysis of accountable care reforms. Health Aff (Millwood) 2017;36(11):1920–7.

48. Tuso P, Huynh DN, Garofalo L, et al. The readmission reduction program of Kaiser Permanente Southern California-knowledge transfer and performance improvement. Perm J 2013;17(3):58–63.

49. Rodin D, Silow-Carroll S. Medicaid payment and delivery reform in Colorado: ACOs at the regional level. The Commonwealth Fund. March 2013. Available at: https://www.commonwealthfund.org/publications/case-study/2013/mar/medicaid-payment-and-delivery-refo rm-colorado-acos-regional-level. Accessed January 7, 2020.

50. Hauptman PJ, Rich MW, Heidenreich PA, et al. The heart failure clinic: a consensus statement of the Heart Failure Society of America. J Card Fail 2008; 14(10):801–15.

51. ClinicalTrials.gov. Bethesda (MD): National Library of Medicine (US). Identifier NCT03334188, Electronic Health Record-leveraged, Patient-centered, Intensification of Chronic Care for HF (EPIC-HF). Available at: https://clinicaltrials.gov/ct2/show/ NCT03334188. Accessed January 4, 2020.

52. Bethesda (MD): National Library of Medicine (US). Identifier NCT03973931, Personalized Patient Data and Behavioral Nudges to Improve Adherence to Chronic Cardiovascular Medications (Nudge) trial. Available at: ClinicalTrials.gov https://clinicaltrials. gov/ct2/show/NCT03973931?term=nudge&draw= 2&rank=7. Accessed January 4, 2020.

53. Gupta N, Kiley ML, Anthony F, et al. Multi-center, community-based cardiac implantable electronic devices registry: population, device utilization, and outcomes. J Am Heart Assoc 2016;5(3):e002798.

54. Piwek L, Ellis DA, Andrews S, et al. The rise of consumer health wearables: promises and barriers. PLoS Med 2016;13(2):e1001953.

55. Kvedar J, Coye MJ, Everett W. Connected health: a review of technologies and strategies to improve patient care with telemedicine and telehealth. Health Aff (Millwood) 2014;33(2):194–9.

56. Smith GH, Shore S, Allen LA, et al. Discussing out-of-pocket costs with patients: shared decision making for sacubitril-valsartan in heart failure. J Am Heart Assoc 2019;8(1):e010635.

57. Knoepke CE, Allen LA, Kramer DB, et al. Medicare mandates for shared decision making in cardiovascular device placement. Circ Cardiovasc Qual Outcomes 2019;12(7):e004899.

58. Centers for Medicare & Medicaid Services. Decision Memo for Percutaneous Left Atrial Appendage (LAA) Closure Therapy (CAG-00445N). 2016. Available at: https://www.cms.gov/medicare-coverage-database/ details/nca-decision-memo.aspx?NCAId=281. Accessed January 8, 2020.

59. Centers for Medicare & Medicaid Services. Decision Memo for Implantable Cardioverter Defibrillators (CAG-00157R4). 2018. Available at: https://www.cms.gov/medicare-coverage-database/ details/nca-decision-memo.aspx?NCAId=288. Accessed January 8, 2020.

60. Psotka MA, Fonarow GC, Allen LA, et al. The hospital readmissions reduction program: nationwide perspectives and recommendations: A JACC: Heart Failure Position Paper. JACC Heart Fail 2020;8(1): 1–11.

61. Next Steps in Measuring Quality of Care in Medicare. Available at: MedPAC.gov http://www.medpac.gov/ docs/default-source/reports/chapter-8-next-steps-in-measuring-quality-of-care-in-medicare-june-2015-report-.pdf?sfvrsn=0. Accessed January 14, 2020.

62. Garvin JH, Kim Y, Gobbel GT, et al. Automating quality measures for heart failure using natural language processing: a descriptive study in the department of veterans affairs. JMIR Med Inform 2018;6(1):e5.

Defragmenting Heart Failure Care
Medical Records Integration

Thomas F. Byrd IV, MD[a],*, Faraz S. Ahmad, MD, MS[b,c],
David M. Liebovitz, MD[d], Abel N. Kho, MD[e,f]

KEYWORDS

- Interoperability • Fragmented • EHR • Electronic health record • Regulation • Data • Informatics
- ONC

KEY POINTS

- Fragmented heart failure care occurs when providers make clinical decisions in the setting of incomplete information.
- Electronic health information exchange is accelerating, driven by federal regulations and evolving data standards.
- New heart failure technologies capture valuable patient-generated data but will not improve care fragmentation in isolation.

INTRODUCTION

The enormous public health burden of heart failure (HF) continues to grow. Between 2009 and 2016, the number of patients living with HF in the United States grew by an estimated 5.7 million.[1] The prevalence of HF is projected to increase by 46% between 2012 and 2030, affecting nearly 3 out of every 100 Americans.[2] It is projected that in 2030, the total annual cost of HF in the United States will amount to $69.8 billion or $244 for every adult.[2] The burden of HF is compounded by high rates of rehospitalizations,[3] driven in part by a lack of transitional care systems that can meet the complex medical needs of patients with HF.[4] Accordingly, a major barrier to delivering the best care for patients with HF is the fragmentation of their health care experience.

Fragmentation refers to dealing in individual parts rather than the whole.[5] Patients who receive care in many different health care settings are exposed to unnecessary medical procedures[6] and diagnostic tests.[7] Patients with fragmented

[a] Department of Medicine (Hospital Medicine), Northwestern University Feinberg School of Medicine, 200 East Ontario Street, Suite 700, Chicago, IL 60611, USA; [b] Department of Medicine (Cardiology), Center for Health Information Partnerships, Institute for Public Health and Medicine, Northwestern University Feinberg School of Medicine, 676 North Saint Clair, Suite 600, Chicago, IL 60611, USA; [c] Department of Preventive Medicine (Health and Biomedical Informatics), Center for Health Information Partnerships, Institute for Public Health and Medicine, Northwestern University Feinberg School of Medicine, 676 North Saint Clair, Suite 600, Chicago, IL 60611, USA; [d] Department of Medicine (General Internal Medicine and Geriatrics), Center for Health Information Partnerships, Institute for Public Health and Medicine, Northwestern University Feinberg School of Medicine, 675 North Street Clair, Suite 18-200, Chicago, IL 60611, USA; [e] Department of Medicine (General Internal Medicine and Geriatrics), Center for Health Information Partnerships, Institute for Public Health and Medicine, Northwestern University Feinberg School of Medicine, 750 North Lake Shore, 10th Floor, Chicago, IL 60611, USA; [f] Department of Preventive Medicine (Health and Biomedical Informatics), Center for Health Information Partnerships, Institute for Public Health and Medicine, Northwestern University Feinberg School of Medicine, 750 North Lake Shore, 10th Floor, Chicago, IL 60611, USA
* Corresponding author.
E-mail address: thomas.byrd@northwestern.edu
Twitter: @freebyrdmd (T.F.B.); @FarazA_MD (F.S.A.)

Heart Failure Clin 16 (2020) 467–477
https://doi.org/10.1016/j.hfc.2020.06.007

care also experience longer hospital stays,[8] whereas patients with better continuity of care have fewer preventable HF hospitalizations.[9] In a fragmented model, care decisions are made by multiple independent providers who have limited means of transmitting information between themselves.

For example, several trials have consistently shown improved outcomes among patients with HF with diabetes who are treated with a sodium/glucose cotransporter 2 (SGLT2) inhibitor.[10–12] In the near future, indications for these medications may expand to nondiabetic patients with HF.[13] Prescribing them necessitates ongoing monitoring for efficacy and side effects, which requires close communication with other providers.[14] Specifically, patients starting an SGLT2 inhibitor should be counseled on the risks of hypoglycemia and volume depletion and may need titration of their antiglycemic medications and diuretics. This task represents a significant care coordination challenge for patients who are simultaneously managed by multiple providers (their primary care clinician, cardiologist, nephrologist, endocrinologist, etc.). If these patients are hospitalized and their HF medications are put on hold or decreased in dose during an admission, determining which provider is responsible for restarting which medication on discharge requires expedient health information transfer and communication. Ideally, to defragment HF care, providers must be able to (1) quickly and easily access all available patient health information and (2) instantaneously have their own management decisions known to the patient and all other treating providers, regardless of location or specialty.

Goals of this Review

In this review, the authors explore why defragmenting HF care through the exchange of health information in the electronic health record (EHR) era has proved to be a persistent and complex challenge. Their discussion on initiatives related to improving care fragmentation focuses on the regulatory landscape that drove EHR adoption and now aims to democratize data access to improve patient care. In addition, the authors explain the central role that data standards and record linkage play within the realm of health information exchange and interoperability as it pertains to patients with HF. Finally, the authors discuss new information technology priorities for HF that are poised to allow patient-generated data to be collected and integrated into clinical decision-making.

INITIATIVES RELATED TO CARE FRAGMENTATION

The advent of the EHR engendered the hope that clinical information would no longer be trapped in a paper chart and instead would be digitally accessible at the moment of medical decision-making. Free-flowing health information exchange between clinics and hospitals, unbounded by geography, would reduce medical errors, adverse events, and costs.[15] Instead, EHR adoption has been characterized by a myriad of competing vendors and noncommunicative software systems, so that missing clinical information outside one's specific practice site remains common.[16] This phenomenon, a key driver of fragmented care, is known as a *lack of interoperability*.

Interoperability defines the capacity of disparate health information technology (IT) systems or devices to exchange, interpret, and make available shared data without special effort on the part of the user.[17] Without interoperability, clinically useful health information exchange is dramatically impaired and care fragmentation soars. Nevertheless, implementing interoperable health IT solutions to defragment HF care has been riddled with challenges that are only now beginning to improve through dedicated regulatory policy and stakeholder alignment.

Regulation

Incentivizing electronic health record adoption
President George W. Bush catalyzed the federal government's involvement in national health IT with his signing of Executive Order 13,335 in 2004 (**Table 1**). Intended to "provide leadership for the development and nationwide implementation of an interoperable health technology infrastructure," the Order established the Office of the National Coordinator for Health Information Technology (ONC), within the US Department of Health and Human Services.[18] Although the ONC mission statement and priorities have evolved over time, its central role in the uptake and regulation of EHR products was cemented through congressional mandate in 2009 as part of the Health Information Technology for Economic and Clinical Health (HITECH) Act.

HITECH provided financial rewards for achieving meaningful use of EHR platforms, intended to encourage the use of health IT above and beyond a basic implementation. With its primary intent being to bring the entire US health system into the digital era, less emphasis was placed on ensuring interoperability of the new software systems—only a 10% electronic transmittal rate of a summary of care document during a patient

Table 1
Summary of legislative efforts to reduce health care fragmentation through information technology

Legislation	President	Year	Health IT Component	Intended Effect
Executive Order 13,335	George W. Bush	2004	Established the Office of the National Coordinator for Health Information Technology (ONC)	Provide leadership for the development of a nationwide health technology infrastructure
Health Information Technology for Economic and Clinical Health (HITECH) Act	Barack Obama	2009	Set meaningful use requirements for adoption of ONC-certified EHRs; tied to Medicaid incentive payments	Encourage use of EHRs to achieve significant improvements in patient care
Affordable Care Act (ACA)	Barack Obama	2010	Established the Hospital Readmission Reduction Program (HRRP); tied to Medicare reimbursement payments	Reduce the prevalence and cost of hospital readmissions nationwide to reduce health care spending
Medicare Access and CHIP Reauthorization Act (MACRA)	Barack Obama	2015	Established the Quality Payment Program (QPP); adjusts Medicare payments based on quality and use of ONC-certified interoperable EHRs	Reward quality of care over fee-for-service; reward use of interoperable health IT
21st Century Cures Act	Barack Obama	2016	Mandates interoperability through health IT regulations and prohibits information blocking	Advance interoperability and support the access, exchange, and use of electronic health information

transfer was required to meet the meaningful use requirement.[19] Although HITECH was successful in stimulating the shift from paper charts to EHRs for most of the hospitals and clinics, any resultant association between EHR adoption and improved patient outcomes remained questionable.[20] Among ambulatory patients with HF, the differences in rates of guideline-directed medical therapy (GDMT) between outpatient cardiology practices using paper charts versus those using an EHR were small and inconsistent.[21] Patients admitted for HF to hospitals using EHRs fared no better than their counterparts at paper-based hospitals with respect to HF quality metrics, readmissions, and mortality.[22]

Reducing readmission reimbursements

In 2010, the Patient Protection and Affordable Care Act became law. The 3 major provisions of the Affordable Care Act included health insurance regulation, insurance expansion, and health delivery system reform. The latter was meant to prioritize quality of care over quantity of care. One way the law aimed to achieve these quality gains was through cuts to the Centers for Medicare and Medicaid Services reimbursement rates for hospitals with higher-than-expected 30-day readmission rates. The initiative, known as the Hospital Readmission Reduction Program, began penalizing hospitals starting in 2013 for readmissions of patients with a selection of common conditions including chronic obstructive pulmonary disease, pneumonia, hip or knee replacement, acute myocardial infarction, and HF. Of these, the most commonly readmitted patients were (and still remain) those with HF.

For patients who are readmitted after a HF hospitalization, fragmentation of care is associated with worse outcomes. Those readmitted to a different hospital than that of their index admission generally experience longer stays and higher mortality risk than those readmitted to the same hospital.[23] Although there may be multiple institutional and situational variables driving this association, a lack of universal medical records integration is a likely contributor. With disparate institutions using different EHRs, none of which were designed to "talk" to each other, interinstitutional health information exchange has traditionally been sparse and unincentivized. To address this deficit, lawmakers introduced new legislation designed to spur EHR interoperability under the growing regulatory auspices of the Office of the National Coordinator for Health Information Technology (ONC).

Mandating interoperability

The Medicare Access and CHIP Reauthorization Act of 2015 created a new incentive program called the Quality Payment Program (QPP) that rewards quality of care and phases out the traditional fee-for-service reimbursement model. Within the QPP, the Merit-based Incentive Payment System adjusts provider payments based on performance within 4 categories. The quality category, as it relates to patients with HF, measures and adjusts for functional outcomes, readmissions, and the percentage of patients prescribed GDMT.[24] The promotion of interoperability category awards points for ONC-certified EHR use demonstrating (without minimal use thresholds) the capabilities of e-prescribing, electronic referral, patient access to health information, and clinical data exchange.[25] Given the recent implementation of these programs, few data are available to judge their effects on HF patient care or outcomes.

In 2016, the 21st Century Cures Act was passed, which tasked the ONC with bolstering interoperability and stimulating health information exchange through mandates that (1) define interoperability, (2) prevent information blocking, (3) develop data sharing standards, and (4) call for Application Programming Interfaces (APIs) that allow patients to access their health information without special effort.[26] An API is a communication tool that allows one computer program to talk to another and request data in a very efficient way; APIs are used in countless mobile apps and software programs that download data from the Internet. Deciphering the potential effects of these types of federal IT regulations on fragmented HF care requires an understanding of the different types of health information exchange that currently exist.

Health Information Exchange

Interoperability allows for health information exchange, which is the electronic access and transmittal of a patient's vital medical information.[27] Participants in health information exchange may include physicians, nurses, caregivers, pharmacists, and any others that have cared, are caring, or will care for that patient, in addition to patients themselves. The ONC has defined 3 specific types of health information exchange, each distinguished by a specific clinical workflow and direction of information transfer (**Fig. 1**).[27]

Directed exchange

First, a directed exchange refers to health information sent over the Internet in a secure fashion, encrypted and reliably transmitted (see **Fig. 1**A). Senders and receivers generally have a preexisting relationship, and information is sent in anticipation of need or by request between individuals. Directed exchange at its simplest might be a primary care physician sending a patient's past medical history to a consulting cardiologist by means of encrypted email.

Query-based exchange

Second, a query-based exchange refers to health information that is available at all times for providers to query when needed (see **Fig. 1**B). This type of exchange is more helpful than a directed exchange for unplanned medical care such as emergency department visits where quick information retrieval is imperative to guide clinical decision-making. Ideally, information from a query-based exchange would be seamlessly integrated into the clinician's workflow and relevant data uploaded the moment a new patient's chart is opened. Unfortunately, the availability and reliability of query-based exchanges has been limited by competing business motivations. Although there have been a few successfully formed health information exchanges in certain states with geographically linked care networks, most of the health care institutions remain wary of sharing valuable patient data without a clear value proposition or regulatory requirement to do so.[28]

Consumer-mediated exchange

Third, a consumer-mediated exchange refers to health information that is owned by and personally curated by patients themselves (see **Fig. 1**C). Patients might review their data for missing or inaccurate details, and they have the ability and responsibility to transfer that information to their care team at the appropriate time. This type of health information exchange is classically compared with online banking, where customers are able to securely track, send, and receive their currency on the Internet and through interoperable Automated Teller Machines across the country.

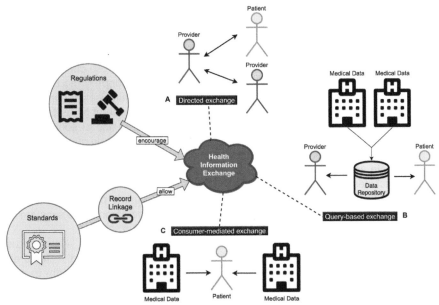

Fig. 1. Models of health information exchange. (*Green arrows*) Legislation tied to health provider reimbursement motivates the use of interoperable health IT; agreed-upon data standards and record linkage provide the framework to securely transmit digitized health information. (*Thin arrows*) Direction of information exchange. (*A*) *Directed exchange*: participants directly send clinical information to and from each other. (*B*) *Query-based exchange*: multiple data sources (ie, patient data from different hospitals) are stored in a repository that users can request specific information from. (*C*) *Consumer-mediated exchange*: health data are collected and stored by the patient who controls who uses the data.

Early attempts to encourage consumer-mediated exchange were met with failure. Google Health, introduced in 2008, offered a centralized service where customers could volunteer their health records from different providers and have them stored in one easily accessible online repository. Adoption among the general population was low, and Google canceled the program in 2012. In parallel, Microsoft introduced its similarly structured HealthVault in 2007, highlighting its ability to collect medical device data such as step counts from fitness monitors and readings from integrated home blood pressure cuffs to generate personalized health insights. After a protracted struggle with poor adoption, HealthVault was discontinued in 2019. In retrospect, the failures of these consumer-mediated exchanges can be partially blamed on a lack of universally agreed-upon standards for sharing health data.[29]

Standards

A standard refers to an idea or an object that others are compared with for purposes of compatibility and consistency. Applied to health information exchange, standards represent agreed-upon ways of using computer code to record and digitally transmit medical information so that the recipient knows exactly what information is present and can translate the code back into a piece of medical information. Google Health and HealthVault relied on poorly adopted and implemented standards such as the Continuity of Care Record that resulted in long, complicated documents that were challenging for both machines and humans to read.[30] As a result, users of these and other early consumer-mediated exchanges ended up with disorganized and unwieldy personal health records.

EHR vendors also rely on standards to comply with interoperability laws. For example, Epic Systems Corporation's Care Everywhere interoperability platform includes data from the Consolidated Clinical Document Architecture standard to allow for point-to-point transfer of health information during transitions of care (thereby satisfying meaningful use requirements).[31] Although widely adopted, this standard also produces a lengthy document containing a potentially vast amount of longitudinal patient data that is difficult for humans to read. Given the usability challenges that arise when too much clinical information is presented at once, the health IT community has gravitated toward a promising new standard: Fast Healthcare Interoperability Resources (FHIR).

Substitutable medical apps, reusable technology on fast healthcare interoperability resources

Fast Healthcare Interoperability Resources (FHIR) was developed by a non-for-profit group called Health Level Seven International (HL7), a standards-development organization focused on the exchange, integration, sharing, and retrieval of electronic health information. As an improvement on prior efforts, FHIR aims for ease of implementation while ensuring consistency and modularity in how data are represented and presented to both machines and humans. In line with the 21st Century Cures Act that stipulates all EHRs must provide APIs to promote health information exchange, FHIR-formatted EHR data are easily accessible through the FHIR API.

On top of the FHIR standard, the app development community SMART (Substitutable Medical Apps, Reusable Technology) coded a technology layer around FHIR that makes it easier to develop FHIR-based apps. Apps that manage data using the FHIR standard with SMART technology are called SMART on FHIR apps. Instead of requesting and then sifting through vast piles of health information, users of SMART on FHIR apps can quickly request a specific piece or set of data, as their most recent medication list, constructed and verified through EHR and pharmacy record data.[29]

Although early efforts at broad adoption of personal health records stumbled, Apple is now generating excitement around Apple Health. Apple Health is a patient-facing, SMART on FHIR app that quickly produces an integrated view of medical record details selectively extracted from multiple EHRs. Patients can elect to share this information with their providers, researchers, or other apps designed to help manage their disease (**Fig. 2**D). In addition, SMART on FHIR apps can be customized to directly appear within the EHR, prepopulated with individualized patient information and displayed via external links, embedded windows, or pop-ups. For example, Schleyer and colleagues[32] have developed an SMART on FHIR app called *Chest Pain Dashboard* that searches the statewide clinical data repository for a patient's prior cardiac studies and presents that information within an EHR window to emergency department physicians caring for patients with chest pain. Their preliminary results show promising reductions in the number of clicks and minutes spent searching for relevant information as compared with their EHR vendor's more cumbersome interoperability platform. Whether SMART on FHIR will improve patient outcomes remains to be seen.

Individual health record linkage

As important as which data are exchanged is whose data are exchanged. Reliable identification of the same patient across care settings remains an incompletely solved challenge. Although some countries have adopted the use of a universal ID for health care purposes,[33] current US regulations prohibit use of federal funds to develop a unique patient identifier. Use of social security numbers (SSNs) as a proxy unique identifier has proved challenging for a variety of reasons, including fraudulent use and diminishing capture of full SSNs at registration.[34] In the absence of a unique identifier, a variety of linkage methods to match patient records across care sites are in use or under development today.

Deterministic record linkage uses exact matches of patient-specific features (eg, first name, last name, date of birth) to assert that records are the same. Probabilistic matching, pioneered through work at the US Census Bureau, uses patient-specific features alongside common or similar variants to create a probability score for a match. Depending on the use case, a threshold level is set above which matches are presumed accurate and below which they are considered nonmatches or require further manual review. Most EHRs and health information exchanges that provide record linkage functionality use probabilistic record linkage methods.

A newer method, referential matching, makes use of additional patient-specific features (eg, voter registration records) to increase match confidence. To reduce the need to share protected health information for matching purposes, privacy preserving record linkage methods use irreversible encryption algorithms to create a unique code for each patient based on available features, and only this encrypted code is shared for generating matches.[35] Regardless of the matching method, the availability and quality of patient-specific features contribute substantially to match quality.[36] Record linkage methods and novel technologies adapted to matching (eg, biometrics) will continue to evolve and play a crucial role in achieving interoperability.

CARE FRAGMENTATION PRIORITIES FOR HEART FAILURE MANAGEMENT
Medication Management

Beyond driving EHR-based information exchange, interoperability gains may improve our ability to capture and transmit data generated outside the hospital. For example, outpatient medical management therapy (pharmacist-led comprehensive medication review, treatment plan formulation,

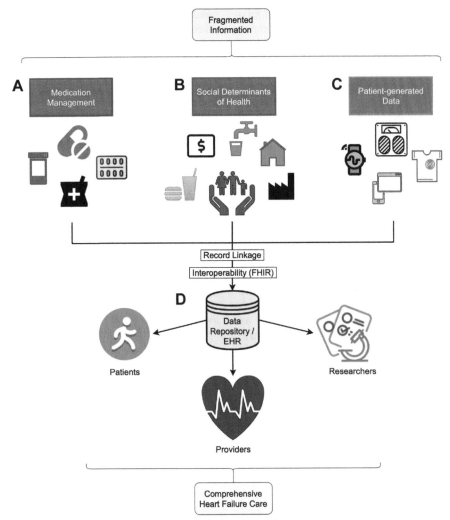

Fig. 2. Comprehensive heart failure care requires interoperability between fragmented data sources. (*A*) *Medication management* data include prescription information, refill history, insurance copay, and pharmacist documentation. (*B*) *Social determinants of health* include patient-reported and census-derived information on poverty, insurance status, food available, living environment, and community resources. (*C*) *Patient-generated data* include readings from home scales or blood pressure cuffs, sensor data from wearable devices such as watches, data from implantable cardiac devices, and information entered through Web portal and smartphone apps. (*D*) These data can be transmitted through FHIR resources to a central database or EHR where they can be used by patients, researchers, and health care providers.

and patient education) has been included in Medicare Part D since 2013, but all documentation is done on paper in isolation from the EHR, rarely finding its way back to prescribers.[37,38] Proponents of FHIR can imagine an app that links medical management therapy data from pharmacy databases to the EHR so that actionable alerts for a specific patient can be routed to the care team or prescriber's inbox (**Fig. 2**A).[39] In this way, a patient with HF seen by a pharmacist for medication review and found to be on suboptimal GDMT doses would instantaneously have this information delivered to the clinical team. Similarly,

Surescripts has developed an SMART on FHIR app that transfers prescription refill history directly into the EHR workflow and outputs an estimated proportion of days covered, allowing clinicians to identify nonadherences issues early on.[40]

Social Determinants of Health

Some of the most important patient health data are external to the health care setting. Social determinants of health (SDOH) are the extrinsic, overlapping social constructs and economic systems that can lead to poor clinical outcomes and include inadequate housing, food, social support, transportation, physical environment, and insurance coverage (**Fig. 2**B). The importance of SDOH in HF care has been validated by the 2019 American Heart Association/American College of Cardiology Guideline on the Primary Prevention of Cardiovascular Disease, which acknowledges that "failure to address the impact of social determinants of health impedes efficacy of proven prevention recommendations."[41] Deriving robust patient-specific treatment plans based on SDOH requires that SDOH data be accurately and comprehensively recorded and addressed. Unfortunately, clinicians often lack the time and resources to document and meaningfully consider these complex issues.[42] Instead, patients typically are screened using pre-visit surveys that ask about basic social determinants (such as intimate partner violence, financial strain, and education level) to satisfy federal requirements for SDOH documentation within the EHR. Some health groups have also added community-level social determinants such as Census Bureau rates of poverty and unemployment into their EHRs for providers to view.[43] Although the emphasis on SDOH documentation has increased the amount of information captured, clinicians have not settled on what to do with it, opening the space for vendor solutions. Now-Pow[44] is one example of a company that leverages FHIR resources to securely integrate SDOH into routine care for the purpose of connecting patients to the most personally relevant community resources.

Home-Based Monitoring

At home daily weights for patients with HF are notoriously difficult for physicians to track and act on, as the onus has traditionally been put on the patient to log these values accurately and report them in a timely fashion. As discussed earlier in the context of failed consumer-mediated exchanges, many patients are not willing or are unable to manage their own health data, including self-generated data such as daily weights. Learning from the challenges of Google Health and Microsoft HealthVault, new health IT companies have found solutions that combine the tenets of consumer-mediated exchange (where the patient generates and stores data) with query-based exchange (where that stored data can be viewed remotely by providers), as depicted in **Fig. 2**C. For example, Rimidi used an SMART on FHIR app to allow connected home scales to securely transmit data to an EHR dashboard that alerts providers to rapid weight gain.[45] Taken to the next level, performing advanced

analytics on this type of data could deliver personalized clinical decision support for diuretic dosing to prevent HF deterioration more successfully than generalized weight thresholds.[46]

Implantable Device Monitoring

Based on the concept of closely monitoring volume status to prevent HF rehospitalizations, the CardioMEMS implantable device was approved in 2014 by the Food and Drug Administration for wireless pulmonary artery pressure monitoring in New York Heart Association class III patients with HF.[47] The European Society of Cardiology lists CardioMEMS implantation as a class IIb, level B recommendation that "may be considered … to reduce the risk of recurrent HF hospitalization,"[48] consistent with before-and-after and matched cohort studies that have demonstrated impressive reductions in HF hospitalizations among patients who received a CardioMEMS device.[49,50] Although some have raised concerns about the real-world applicability of these studies,[51] having continuous intravascular pulmonary artery pressure and heart rate data available to guide HF care seems to be useful for a subset of patients with HF. Unfortunately, obtaining this information is also a fragmented process. Clinicians must log on to an external, proprietary Web portal to view patient device data and are instructed to rely on email alerts for notifications of impending patient crisis. Finding and accessing these data can be prohibitively difficult for inpatient physicians without CardioMEMS platform knowledge who might otherwise act on these data to deliver improved care during an HF hospitalization. Developing ways to integrate these types of device-generated data into the EHR using tools such as SMART on FHIR would represent a powerful step toward individualized, defragmented HF care (see **Fig. 2**D).[52]

DISCUSSION

HF continues to grow in prevalence and care complexity. Robust clinical trials have generated high-quality, evidence-based recommendations and guidelines shown to improve quality of life and mortality. Paradoxically, the more GDMTs that emerge, the more fragmented patient care can become. Comprehensively treating the whole patient, including comorbid conditions and social determinants of health, often requires the addition of more care providers and more detailed management plans. Frequent hospitalizations and readmissions compound the fragmented care that patient with HF receives.

Because care coordination requires clinical data, early efforts to defragment care were focused on legislation to encourage EHR adoption, assuming that digitized data inherently would be more accessible to providers than paper charts. Clinicians quickly realized that computerized data alone were not enough; rather, health information had to be quickly and easily transferrable. Health information exchange through interoperability has become the new goal for those wanting to improve the quality of HF care delivery. Motivated by legislative mandates, improved standards such as FHIR are being adopted to allow for fast and succinct clinical data transfer.

In response to the Hospital Readmissions Reduction Program incentivizing reduced HF readmissions, vendors have created a plethora of novel solutions for capturing patient-generated data that might warn of impending decompensation. Each of these solutions, whether it be a WiFi-enabled home scale or an implantable cardiac device, runs the risk of perpetuating fragmented care if its data remain siloed outside of the patient's health record and inaccessible by the care team.

Although legislative efforts to improve secure health information exchange continue to evolve, advocating for interoperability and patient access to data should remain a top priority for the HF providers. Companies that benefit from control over access to data, including EHR vendors, can impede efforts to defragment care, and regulation intended to support interoperability may help offset this self-interest. Above all, patients should be the ones who benefit the most from their electronically collected health information—achieving the rapid, seamless exchange of these data is key to realizing health care improvements in the EHR era.

DISCLOSURE

A.N. Kho is an advisor to Datavant. D.M. Liebovitz has ownership equity and is an advisor to Bedside Intelligence, LLC, and Optima Integrated Health. The other authors have nothing to disclose.

REFERENCES

1. Benjamin Emelia J, Paul M, Alonso A, et al. Heart disease and stroke statistics—2019 update: a report from the American Heart Association. Circulation 2019;139(10):e56–528.
2. Heidenreich PA, Albert NM, Allen LA, et al. Forecasting the impact of heart failure in the United States: a policy statement from the American Heart Association. Circ Heart Fail 2013;6(3):606–19.
3. Kilgore M, Patel HK, Kielhorn A, et al. Economic burden of hospitalizations of Medicare beneficiaries with heart failure. Risk Manag Healthc Policy 2017; 10:63–70.
4. Allen Larry A, Fonarow Gregg C, Liang Li, et al. Medication initiation burden required to comply with heart failure guideline recommendations and hospital quality measures. Circulation 2015; 132(14):1347–53.
5. Stange KC. The problem of fragmentation and the need for integrative solutions. Ann Fam Med 2009; 7(2):100–3.
6. Romano MJ, Segal JB, Pollack CE. The association between continuity of care and the overuse of medical procedures. JAMA Intern Med 2015;175(7): 1148–54.
7. Kern LM, Seirup JK, Casalino LP, et al. Healthcare fragmentation and the frequency of radiology and other diagnostic tests: a cross-sectional study. J Gen Intern Med 2017;32(2):175–81.
8. Galanter WL, Applebaum A, Boddipalli V, et al. Migration of patients between five urban teaching hospitals in Chicago. J Med Syst 2013;37(2):9930.
9. Nyweide DJ, Anthony DL, Bynum JPW, et al. Continuity of care and the risk of preventable hospitalization in older adults. JAMA Intern Med 2013;173(20): 1879–85.
10. Neal B, Perkovic V, Mahaffey KW, et al. Canagliflozin and cardiovascular and renal events in type 2 diabetes. N Engl J Med 2017;377(7):644–57.
11. Wiviott SD, Raz I, Bonaca MP, et al. Dapagliflozin and cardiovascular outcomes in type 2 diabetes. N Engl J Med 2019;380(4):347–57.
12. Zinman B, Wanner C, Lachin JM, et al. Empagliflozin, cardiovascular outcomes, and mortality in type 2 diabetes. N Engl J Med 2015;373(22):2117–28.
13. McMurray JJV, Solomon SD, Inzucchi SE, et al. Dapagliflozin in patients with heart failure and reduced ejection fraction. N Engl J Med 2019;381(21): 1995–2008.
14. Vardeny O, Vaduganathan M. Practical guide to prescribing sodium-glucose cotransporter 2 inhibitors for cardiologists. JACC Heart Fail 2019;7(2):169–72.
15. Bourgeois FC, Olson KL, Mandl KD. Patients treated at multiple acute health care facilities: quantifying information fragmentation. Arch Intern Med 2010; 170(22):1989–95.
16. Smith PC, Araya-Guerra R, Bublitz C, et al. Missing clinical information during primary care visits. JAMA 2005;293(5):565–71.
17. Interoperability | HealthIT.gov. Available at: https://www.healthit.gov/topic/interoperability. Accessed January 10, 2020.
18. Incentives for the use of health information technology and establishing the position of the national

health information technology coordinator. Federal register. Available at: https://www.federalregister.gov/documents/2004/04/30/04-10024/incentives-for-the-use-of-health-information-technology-and-establishing-the-position-of-the. Accessed January 7, 2020.

19. Medicare and Medicaid Programs; Electronic health record incentive program-stage 3 and modifications to meaningful use in 2015 through 2017. Federal register. Available at: https://www.federalregister.gov/documents/2015/10/16/2015-25595/medicare-and-medicaid-programs-electronic-health-record-incentive-program-stage-3-and-modifications. Accessed January 7, 2020.

20. Halamka JD, Tripathi M. The HITECH era in retrospect. N Engl J Med 2017;377(10):907–9.

21. Walsh MN, Yancy CW, Albert NM, et al. Electronic health records and quality of care for heart failure. Am Heart J 2010;159(4):635–42.e1.

22. Senthil S, Fonarow Gregg C, Sheng S, et al. Association of electronic health record use with quality of care and outcomes in heart failure: an analysis of get with the guidelines—heart failure. J Am Heart Assoc 2018;7(7):e008158.

23. McAlister Finlay A, Erik Y, Kaul Pa. Patients with heart failure readmitted to the original hospital have better outcomes than those readmitted elsewhere. J Am Heart Assoc 2017;6(5):e004892.

24. Wolfe JD, Joynt Maddox KE. Heart failure and the affordable care act: past, present, and future. JACC Heart Fail 2019;7(9):737–45.

25. MIPS. Promoting Interoperability (PI). Available at: https://www.aafp.org/practice-management/payment/medicare-payment/mips/aci.html. Accessed January 9, 2020.

26. 21st Century Cures Act: Interoperability, Information Blocking, and the ONC Health IT Certification Program. Federal Register. 2019. Available at: https://www.federalregister.gov/documents/2019/03/04/2019-02224/21st-century-cures-act-interoperability-information-blocking-and-the-onc-health-it-certification. Accessed January 9, 2020.

27. What is HIE? | HealthIT.gov. Available at: https://www.healthit.gov/topic/health-it-and-health-information-exchange-basics/what-hie. Accessed January 9, 2020.

28. Mahajan AP. Health information exchange—obvious choice or pipe dream? JAMA Intern Med 2016;176(4):429–30.

29. Braunstein ML. Health care in the age of interoperability part 5: the personal health record. IEEE Pulse 2019;10(3):19–23.

30. Ferranti JM, Musser RC, Kawamoto K, et al. The clinical document architecture and the continuity of care record: a critical analysis. J Am Med Inform Assoc 2006;13(3):245–52.

31. Epic interoperability Fact sheet. Available at: https://www.healthit.gov/sites/default/files/facas/GSG_TestimonySupport_CarlDvorak_2014-08-15_04.pdf. Accessed February 5, 2020.

32. Schleyer TKL, Rahurkar S, Baublet AM, et al. Preliminary evaluation of the Chest Pain Dashboard, a FHIR-based approach for integrating health information exchange information directly into the clinical workflow. AMIA Jt Summits Transl Sci Proc 2019;2019:656–64.

33. Nøhr C, Parv L, Kink P, et al. Nationwide citizen access to their health data: analysing and comparing experiences in Denmark, Estonia and Australia. BMC Health Serv Res 2017;17(1):534.

34. Culbertson A, Goel S, Madden MB, et al. The building blocks of interoperability. a multisite analysis of patient demographic attributes available for matching. Appl Clin Inform 2017;8(2):322–36.

35. Kho AN, Cashy JP, Jackson KL, et al. Design and implementation of a privacy preserving electronic health record linkage tool in Chicago. J Am Med Inform Assoc 2015;22(5):1072–80.

36. Grannis SJ, Xu H, Vest JR, et al. Evaluating the effect of data standardization and validation on patient matching accuracy. J Am Med Inform Assoc 2019;26(5):447–56.

37. Adeoye OA, Farley JF, Coe AB, et al. Medication therapy management delivery by community pharmacists: Insights from a national sample of Medicare Part D beneficiaries. J Am Coll Clin Pharm 2019;2(4):373–82.

38. Brandt NJ, Cooke CE, Sharma K, et al. Findings from a national survey of medicare beneficiary perspectives on the medicare part D medication therapy management standardized format. J Manag Care Spec Pharm 2019;25(3):366–91.

39. Bosworth HB, Zullig LL, Mendys P, et al. Health information technology: meaningful use and next steps to improving electronic facilitation of medication adherence. JMIR Med Inform 2016;4(1):e9.

40. Medication Adherence Solution for Clinicians & PBMs | Surescripts. Available at: https://surescripts.com/inform-care-decisions/insights-alerts/. Accessed January 10, 2020.

41. Arnett DK, Blumenthal RS, Albert MA, et al. 2019 ACC/AHA Guideline on the Primary Prevention of Cardiovascular Disease: A Report of the American College of Cardiology/American Heart Association Task Force on clinical practice guidelines. Circulation 2019;140(11):e596–646.

42. Hammond G, Maddox KEJ. A theoretical framework for clinical implementation of social determinants of health. JAMA Cardiol 2019;4(12):1189–90.

43. Cantor MN, Thorpe L. Integrating data on social determinants of health into electronic health records. Health Aff (Millwood) 2018;37(4):585–90.

44. NowPow. NowPow. Available at: http://wordpress-site.nowpow.com. Accessed January 10, 2020.

45. Rimidi | Solutions. Rimidi. Available at: https://rimidi.com/solutions. Accessed January 10, 2020.

46. Ledwidge MT, O'Hanlon R, Lalor L, et al. Can individualized weight monitoring using the HeartPhone algorithm improve sensitivity for clinical deterioration of heart failure? Eur J Heart Fail 2013;15(4):447–55.

47. Abraham WT, Perl L. Implantable hemodynamic monitoring for heart failure patients. J Am Coll Cardiol 2017;70(3):389–98.

48. Ponikowski P, Voors AA, Anker SD, et al. 2016 ESC Guidelines for the diagnosis and treatment of acute and chronic heart failure: The Task Force for the diagnosis and treatment of acute and chronic heart failure of the European Society of Cardiology (ESC) Developed with the special contribution of the Heart Failure Association (HFA) of the ESC. Eur Heart J 2016;37(27):2129–200.

49. Abraham J, Bharmi R, Jonsson O, et al. Association of ambulatory hemodynamic monitoring of heart failure with clinical outcomes in a concurrent matched cohort analysis. JAMA Cardiol 2019;4(6):556–63.

50. Desai AS, Bhimaraj A, Bharmi R, et al. Ambulatory hemodynamic monitoring reduces heart failure hospitalizations in "real-world" clinical practice. J Am Coll Cardiol 2017;69(19):2357–65.

51. Krumholz HM, Dhruva SS. Real-world data on heart failure readmission reduction: real or real uncertain?*. J Am Coll Cardiol 2017;69(19):2366–8.

52. van der Velde ET, Foeken H, Witteman TA, et al. Integration of data from remote monitoring systems and programmers into the hospital electronic health record system based on international standards. Neth Heart J 2012;20(2):66–70.

Adapting to the Reimbursement Landscape
The Future of Value-Based Care

Jessica Walradt, MS[a], Hannah Alphs Jackson, MD, MHSA[a,b],*

KEYWORDS

- Payment reform • Bundled payments • Alternative payment models • Value-based care

KEY POINTS

- Rising health care costs have created an imperative for the emergence of alternative payment models.
- Heart failure has emerged as a popular target of alternative payment, including the Hospital Readmission Reduction Program (HRRP) and the Bundled Payment for Care Improvement (BPCI) and BPCI Advanced initiatives.
- Translating payment models into clinical care redesign requires (1) an understanding of the target population, (2) the drivers of health care expenditures in that target population, including a detailed understanding of sources of clinical variation, and (3) knowledge of resources and processes that can be aligned as a cohesive intervention to reduce variation in clinical variation.
- Northwestern Medicine's experience in BPCI is used as a case study to illustrate how alternative payment models accelerated redesign of its care delivery for heart failure admissions.

INTRODUCTION

An examination of process improvement in health care would be incomplete without an exploration of one of the undeniable driving forces of behavior: payment. The method in which health care is reimbursed creates a host of opportunities and challenges for the way health care is delivered. Historically, health services have predominantly been reimbursed on a fee-for-service basis, meaning providers receive payment from purchasers of health care for each unique treatment, procedure, and/or device delivered to a patient. In general, if a clinician or medical facility delivers a service, they are guaranteed payment, regardless of the patient's health outcome. This fee-for-service system produces 2 unintended consequences: (1)

providers are incentivized to focus on the volume of services rather than the value of services; and (2) there is little motivation to focus on the longitudinal patient experience, meaning what happens to the patient when they leave a provider's clinic or facility. The system can lead to the provision of fragmented care and unnecessary utilization of health care services.

The belief that if reimbursement is a significant factor in some of the undesired economic challenges facing our health care system today, then *alternative* reimbursement mechanisms can also be a solution, has led economists, insurers, and policy makers to develop alternatives to fee-for-service, often called alternative payment models (APMs). Although a multitude of constructs of an

[a] Department of Managed Care, Northwestern Memorial HealthCare, 541 North Fairbanks Court, Suite 1500, Chicago, IL 60611, USA; [b] Department of Surgery, Feinberg School of Medicine, Northwestern University, Chicago, IL, USA
* Corresponding author. Department of Managed Care, Northwestern Memorial HealthCare, 541 North Fairbanks Court, Suite 1500, Chicago, IL 60611, USA.
E-mail address: hannah.alphsjackson@nm.org
Twitter: @HannahJacksonMD (H.A.J.)

Heart Failure Clin 16 (2020) 479–487
https://doi.org/10.1016/j.hfc.2020.06.008
1551-7136/20/© 2020 Elsevier Inc. All rights reserved.

APM exist, a core commonality is a methodology that incentivizes providers to deliver high-quality and cost-efficient care. APMs can take many forms, from a simple pay-for-performance model in which providers receive bonuses for achieving certain health outcomes, to shared-risk models under which providers may actually lose money if they do not meet certain quality and utilization goals.

In recent years, the prevalence of APMs as the means of reimbursement for health care dollars has increased dramatically. Each year, the Health Care Payment and Learning Action Network surveys insurers to assess what percentage of their reimbursement is paid through APMs versus traditional fee-for-service. In 2015, approximately 38% of health care dollars were paid through APMs. In 2018, this figure grew to 60%.[1] This article explores common types of APMs, the factors that necessitated the creation of APMs, the forces leading to recent increases in the prevalence of these payment models, and how APMs can drive clinical process improvement and clinical care redesign using a clinical case study.

Common Forms of Alternative Payment Models

APMs create increased incentives for providers to focus on the outcomes related to quality, quantity and appropriateness of services provided to patients. This is achieved by linking the amount of payment received, and ultimately income generated by, health care providers to process and outcome measures and/or the overall amount of services and corresponding costs provided to a patient. APMs differ in terms of their scope (patient population and duration) and the extent to which they shift financial risk from the insurer to the provider (**Table 1**). Some APMs, such as pay-for-performance, simply award provider bonuses or small positive adjustments to their fee schedule payments for surpassing certain process and/or outcome measure thresholds. Other payment mechanisms, such as capitated payments, shift a tremendous amount of risk to providers by only guaranteeing providers a certain per member per month payment based on the patient's risk profile but regardless of actual utilization. Meanwhile, other models like bundled payments provide a middle ground of risk, by applying only to a specific patient group for a time-limited period. Under retrospective bundled payment models, an episode of care is triggered by a diagnosis and/or procedure. An episode can last 30 days, 90 days, or up to 6 months. Providers continue to be reimbursed on a fee-for-service basis throughout the episode, but following the conclusion of an episode

payments for rendered services are summed and compared with a financial target. If payments fall below the target, the bundled payment participant is eligible to receive the difference as savings. However, if payments exceed the target, the participant provider must typically repay the difference back to the insurer as a loss. These types of payment models encourage providers to attempt to manage the totality of a patient's care across time and provider types.

The Origin and Growth of Alternative Payment Models

Health care spending in the United States has grown steadily over the past half century, with total health care expenditures accounting for just 5% of gross domestic product (GDP) in 1960 to 17.7% of the GDP in 2018. During this period, the US population increased in size by 75% while health care expenditures increased by 13,317%.[2,3] Although other nations have also experienced a growth in health expenditures, US health care spending still dramatically outpaces that of other countries. In 2018, the United States spent $3.6 trillion on health care, which amounted to $11,172 per capita. The country with the second-highest per capita health expenditures, Switzerland, spends only approximately $8,000 per capita.[4] This discrepancy becomes more disconcerting when considering the fact that Americans exhibit comparably worse health outcomes in numerous categories when compared with populations of other high-income nations.

Data from the Organization for Economic Cooperation and Development shows that the United States has the lowest life expectancy, the highest infant mortality and maternal mortality, and the highest percentage of overweight or obese adults when compared with 10 other high-income nations.[5] Of course, in many instances US health outcomes were comparably excellent. For example, 30-day mortality for ischemic stroke was 4.2 per 100 patients in the United States compared with a mean of 7.9 per 100 patients in all 11 countries.[5] Still, many academics and policymakers agree that the United States is generating relatively high-quality outcomes commensurate with the level of health care spending.

To understand the connection between this notion and APMs, one must understand the drivers of high health expenditures in the United States. Expenditures are a product of price and utilization; that is, the price paid for health services multiplied by the amount of services provided to the population (**Fig. 1**). The United States' comparably high payment rates are well documented, and often credited to factors such as drug prices, the high

Table 1
Common forms of alternative payment models (APMs)

APM Type	Payment Methodology	Population	Duration	Downside Risk to Provider?	Example
Pay-for-performance	Adjustment to fee schedule based on process and outcome measures	Hospital or provider group-level patients with qualifying encounters	Typically annual	Depends; adjustments can be positive only, negative only, of a combination	Hospital Readmissions Reduction Program
Bundled payments	Payments for services provided to patients reconciled against a target; providers eligible to receive/pay back first dollar savings/losses	Condition or procedure-specific	Typically 90 d (can be 30 d–6 mo)	Typically yes	BPCI Advanced
Accountable care organization (ACO)	Patient service payments reconciled against a benchmark; ACO is eligible to share in savings	Provider group's primary care patients	Annual	Depends; some models only feature shared savings	Pathways to Success
Capitation	Providers receive per member per month payment regardless of actual service utilization	All patients with specific insurance coverage	Annual	Yes	Medicare Advantage

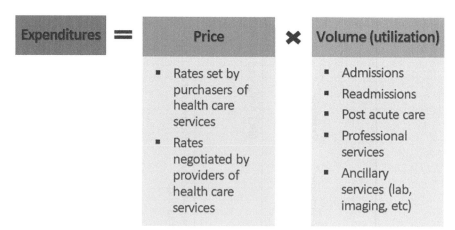

Fig. 1. Key drivers of health care expenditures.

cost of medical training, and excessive administrative costs associated with managing multiple insurance products.[5,6] Drivers of price have been traditionally targeted through absolute reductions in reimbursement rates paid for services (via negotiation or regulatory processes), narrow network design (eg, eliminating higher cost providers or leveraging promises of higher volume for discounted reimbursement rates), and other tactics that are often outside of a clinician's control. These methods can also inadvertently reduce access to care for those who need it most. On the other hand, health systems and clinicians can help impact the second component of total expenditures, utilization, or the quantity (and appropriateness) of services provided.

Not all utilization is necessary, and some utilization can actually be harmful. One strategy for pinpointing potentially unnecessary utilization is to search for examples of variation in the care provided to patients with similar attributes and/or medical conditions. The Dartmouth Atlas Project has spent years reviewing health care spending across regions and unveiled a tremendous amount of variation. For example, in 2008, Dartmouth researchers released annual adjusted per capita Medicare spending figures, and reported a low of $6,264 in Rapid City, South Dakota, and an average high of $15,571 in Miami, Florida.[7] They went on to discover that much of the variation could be explained by differences in inpatient hospitalizations and post-acute care (PAC) utilization. For example, in 2009 the hospital referral region with the lowest heart failure (HF) 30-day readmission rate had a rate of 11.4, whereas the region with the highest readmission rate had a rate of 26.4.[8] A subsequent Dartmouth Atlas study revealed large variation in PAC utilization following surgical procedures between hospitals. For

example, PAC spending post-hospitalization for a total hip replacement varied by 129% between hospitals in the lowest and highest spending quintiles.[9]

Granted, health care costs have been rising steadily for years, and APMs themselves are not a new concept. Diagnosis-related groups (DRGs) are arguably one of the earliest forms of capitation in the United States. From fiscal years 1967 to 1984, hospitals submitted cost reports listing itemized expenditures for Medicare beneficiaries and were paid on the basis of the actual cost.[10] To contain costs, Medicare ultimately switched to a per-case or per-admission reimbursement system in which Medicare paid hospitals a flat rate per case for inpatient hospital care based on the DRG, to incentivize efficiency. In reality, the largest most recent catalyzing factor behind the proliferation APMs is a political one.

In 2009, under the authority of the Medicare Prescription Drug, Improvement, and Modernization Act of 2003, the Centers for Medicare and Medicaid Services (CMS) launched a 3-year demonstration program, the Medicare Acute Episode (ACE) Demonstration, building off the DRG concept and bundling payments episodes of care related to 28 cardiac and 9 orthopedic inpatient surgical services and procedures using a global payment for all Part A and B services, including physician services, pertaining to the inpatient stay for Medicare fee-for-service beneficiaries, in an effort to better align incentives for both hospitals and physicians.[11] Shortly thereafter, in March of 2010, then President Barack Obama signed the Affordable Care Act (ACA) into law. Although the ACA primarily focused on expanding access to health insurance, a small initially overlooked provision of the law would have a massive impact on the reimbursement landscape. Section 3021 established the Center for Medicare and Medicaid Innovation (CMMI), which was charged with designing, implementing, and testing new payment models designed to reduce costs while maintaining or improving the quality of care delivered.[12] Since 2011, CMMI has launched more than 40 APMs, with additional models currently under development. Separate sections of the ACA also provided for the establishment of a pay-for-performance model, the Hospital Readmissions Reduction Program (HRRP), and for the creation of a population-based Medicare Accountable Care Organization (ACO) model through the Medicare Shared Savings Program.[12] The Obama Administration further fueled the momentum created by the ACA when in January 2015, Secretary of Health and Human Services Sylvia Burwell announced the Administration's goal of tying at least 50% of Medicare payments to quality or value by 2018.[13] However, the central question is whether or not these models really can and do incentivize the type of transformation in clinical utilization their designers envision. Contemporary APMs and payment reform efforts, while also designed to ultimately reduce health care expenditures in total, in theory and if well-designed, attempt to align financial incentives in a way that encourages optimal, evidence-based utilization of health care services through clinical redesign.

FINANCIAL MODELS ≠ CARE MODELS: TRANSLATING PAYMENT MODELS INTO CLINICAL CARE REDESIGN OPPORTUNITIES

As articulated previously, it is well understood that health care costs are rising at an unsustainable pace, so it is of no surprise that purchasers of health care, the government, employers, commercial payers, have continued to deploy strategies that both reduce the price paid for health care services as well as reduce the utilization of services, the 2 key drivers of expenditures (see **Fig. 1**). As the single largest payer for health care in the country, Medicare often sets the reimbursement trend for other private purchasers of health care.

A classic target of payment reform efforts, both indirectly and directly, has been the hospital readmission. Whether clinically appropriate or not, a readmission in a purely fee-for-service reimbursement model, is a source of revenue for the care delivery system. In a purely fee-for-service world, there is no financial incentive for a hospital or physician to attempt to monitor and control services provided to their patients beyond the inpatient stay; a hospital is not incentivized to prevent a potential future readmission. APMs in their

variety of forms, seek to create rewards (or disincentives) to make necessary clinical care improvements and redesign to reduce readmissions. The key to payment reform, is therefore not just about the reimbursement schemas. It is how these different financial incentives are translated into tactics to support improvements in the way care is delivered. These improvements may take the form of incremental optimization of existing processes, but can also require investment in structure, people and process to supplement the existing care model, the latter which can create challenges to continuous improvement and other process-focused optimization paradigms.

The ultimate goal of "value-based care" interventions is to achieve the quadruple aim: reduce costs, improve quality outcomes and experience for patients while simultaneously improving the caregiver experience.[14] Although there is likely no singular approach to what has become widely become the clinical transformation of "value-based care," one approach, used successfully at Northwestern Medicine, has been to answer a somewhat stepwise set of questions and considerations in designing population-based approaches. These questions are certainly not exhaustive, nor do they represent the same set of questions that leaders would want to use if deciding to take risk in an alternative model, nor do they address operational feasibility of any given intervention. However, these questions do provide a framework for thinking through implementation of an alternative care model, essentially translating a financial model into digestible and clinically relevant buckets of work.

1. Who is the *target* population, *really*?
2. What are the key *drivers* of health care expenditures in the population?
   - Is there clinical variation?
   - Is that clinical variation "controllable" or "warranted" (vs being the result of a chronic and/or progressive disease process)?
   - For unwarranted clinical variation identified, what are the *causes* of that variation in care delivery *across* the population?
3. Can the source of variation be targeted through an intervention?

CASE STUDY: APPLYING REDESIGN EFFORTS FOR CARE OF CONGESTIVE HEART FAILURE IN THE CENTERS FOR MEDICARE AND MEDICAID'S BUNDLED PAYMENT FOR CARE IMPROVEMENT INITIATIVE

According to data published by the Centers for Disease Control and Prevention and reported by the

American Heart Association, approximately 6.5 million adults in the United States suffer from heart failure.[15,16] In 2012, the cost of health care services, medicines to treat heart failure, and missed days of work cost the nation an estimated $30.7 billion. Data from CMS's Fiscal Year (FY) 2017 Inpatient Utilization and Payment Public Use File (Inpatient PUF), summarizing average payments for the more than 3000 US hospitals that receive Medicare Inpatient Prospective Payment System (IPPS) payments by Medicare Severity DRG (MS-DRG), shows that MS-DRG 291 (HEART FAILURE & SHOCK with major complicating or comorbid condition [MCC]) is the third most common cause of hospital admission for that population, accounting for more than 350,000 inpatient admissions with $3.3 billion in associated Medicare expenditures.[2,3] Across all heart failure–specific MS-DRGs (291 - HEART FAILURE & SHOCK W MCC; 292 - HEART FAILURE & SHOCK with complicating or comorbid condition [CC]; and 293 - HEART FAILURE & SHOCK W/O CC/MCC), heart failure accounts for nearly 500,000 inpatient admissions associated with $4.1 billion in associated Medicare expenditures.[2,3] Based on prevalence and cost in the inpatient setting alone, it is easy to understand why heart failure has been a target for a variety of APMs, including HRRP and CMMI's initial and subsequent versions of the Bundled Payment for Care Improvement (BPCI) initiative and BPCI Advanced (BCPI-A), respectively. Further, heart failure, a chronic disease characterized by acute exacerbations is an area in which therapies, technologies, and standards of care continue to evolve introducing clinical variation in practice as well as creating fragmented delivery between outpatient and inpatient settings as well as between primary care and specialists.

BPCI was (and in current iteration remains in the BPCI-A iteration) a classic example of an episode-based alternative payment model. Essentially, the payment model focused on a defined period of time (30–90 days) an inpatient admission for a particular disease or procedure. In the case of congestive heart failure, 3 different DRGs related to acute care hospital admissions for congestive heart failure were included in the "Congestive Heart Failure" bundle: DRG 291, DRG 292, DRG 293. CMS incentives coordination of care across these episodes of care, and shares savings (or losses), or reductions (or increases) in total health care expenditures across the episode for the population, with providers willing manage the care of the population.

Who Is the Target Population, Really?

In the case of BPCI, the financial model was based on a classification system that is ultimately used for reimbursement, not clinical care delivery. In the case of bundles related to acute exacerbation of chronic disease, patients do not present to the emergency room or to their primary care physician with a DRG. Rather they present with a set of symptoms and, in some cases, a history of certain chronic diseases that provide clues to the acute process. The DRG might be assigned days or even weeks after discharge from the hospital. One study from the Northwestern Medicine Bluhm Cardiovascular Institute demonstrated that between both the 30-day heart failure readmission measure from the HRRP and the DRG-groupings encompassing the BPCI Congestive Heart Failure bundle, fewer than 50% of the population of Medicare patients 65 years or older with actively managed heart failure are captured.[17] Focusing initial efforts and analyses on a DRG-based population might therefore limit the validity, relevance, and clinical appeal of any downstream tactics. Thus, although the financial model is "scored" based on an ultimately different cohort, the care model should focus on clinical interventions that prospectively identify true burden of the disease process, targeting all patients with actively managed heart failure.

This challenge of identifying a target patient population was addressed by using the electronic medical record (EMR)-mined data to enhance the prospective specificity. In other words, rather than relying on MS-DRG billing data to identify patients, as billing data are often available with a lag and only after discharge (not to mention that patients clinically present with symptoms not billing codes), a discrete (and predictive) set of elements about all patients admitted to the hospital (including laboratory values, imaging findings and medication orders), combined with a set of historical diagnoses from prior encounters with the health care system, were mined to produce a highly sensitive (but less specific) patient population list..[18] Daily manual optimization through clinical curation produces a final "list" of probable heart failure admissions across a given facility that supports not only the daily operational workflow, but also the ongoing monitoring of process and outcome metrics in the population. "Identification of Heart Failure Patients in Large Datasets," by Kadosh and colleagues, elsewhere in this issue, also has further information on strategies for identification of heart failure patients.

What Are the Key Drivers of Health Care Expenditures in the Population?

Evaluating total health care expenditures, different from "internal" or health-system specific cost analyses commonly used to derive operating margins and other internal financial metrics, requires comprehensive claims data. Without claims data, using EMR data from a single institution would severely underestimate utilization occurring outside that institution, including readmissions to other hospitals and care delivered in post-acute settings. Therefore, to understand the driver of health care expenditures in the BPCI population, Northwestern Medicine reviewed comprehensive historical claims data provided by Medicare as a component of participation in the BPCI initiative. Each patient's individual expenditures over the duration of the congestive heart failure episode were categorized into a set of distinct groupings: index facility (expenditures related to the heart failure admission that "triggered" the BPCI episode), professional services related to the index admission, readmissions, professional services related to any readmissions, inpatient rehabilitation facility, skilled nursing facility, home health, outpatient facility and professional services, and a few other smaller groupings. For congestive heart failure episodes at Northwestern Memorial Hospital over a period of 18 months evaluated, the clear driver of variation in health care expenditures was readmissions (**Fig. 2**). Readmissions were present in more than half of the episodes and the expenditures related to the episode often exceeded expenditures related to the index admission.

But, what was driving these readmissions? In the Medicare data set used by Northwestern Medicine, prices were normalized. In other words, the variation seen was not caused by differences in prices paid by Medicare to readmissions occurring at different hospitals. The differences in expenditures were a reflection of differences in readmission rates across the population.

Heart failure is usually the result of a chronic and progressive disease process, so the presence of readmissions in and of itself was not an indicator of unwarranted clinical variation. In other words, as patients succumb to disease process, there is some level of expected increase in utilization of health care services. To evaluate whether at least some of the readmission variation observed in the data was "controllable" or "warranted," the Northwestern Medicine team undertook another set of analyses, focused on internal EMR data, to glean patterns. A combination of data mining and comprehensive manual chart review was used, and causes of readmission were identified and categorized as avoidable or unavoidable using internally defined taxonomies. Unanticipated complications (such as a trauma), scheduled procedures or interventions, and biological disease progression were all categorized as unavoidable. Although advances in artificial intelligence, natural language processing, and data mining will no doubt continue to help support, augment, and accelerate these types of analyses, the value of a clinician-driven chart review is in finding patterns that are not immediately coded as discrete data elements. And in the case of the chart review for heart failure readmissions at Northwestern Medicine, many avoidable sources of readmission, not always available in discrete data, were observed: clinical care pathway and discharge protocol compliance, clinical discharge appropriateness, behavioral health factors, barriers to care resulting from social determinants of health, and patient activation were some of the major themes identified.

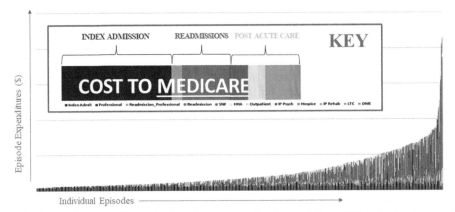

Fig. 2. Individual episode expenditures for Medicare congestive heart failure BPCI episodes over an 18-month period at one of the Northwestern Medicine's acute care hospitals participating in the BPCI program. (©2020 DataGen®, Inc.)

Can the Source of Variation Be Targeted Through an Intervention?

For the heart failure BPCI paradigm, the key underlying questions to support development of a clinically driven, targeted intervention were about (1) ability to identify the target population within 24 hours of admission, (2) the deployment of a multidisciplinary approach for the targeted population in all settings, and (3) the ability to measure the execution of that multidisciplinary approach in near real-time.

Individually and clinically targeted interventions are critical to ensure the appropriate resources are being deployed for the identified needs. In the case of Northwestern Medicine's heart failure population, in response to the multifactorial reasons underlying unwarranted readmissions, a multidisciplinary team, including physicians, advance practice providers, nurses, educators, social work, pharmacy, nutritionists, and behavioral health providers were developed to support inpatient care and transition to outpatient care. Early data demonstrate that, for instance, for patients with complex medication regimens or patients who have changes in their inpatient medication regimens, pharmacist-led transitions of care telephone calls identify and reduce medication errors in heart failure patients post-discharge.[19]

Timely follow-up in clinic after heart failure hospitalization represents another important lever for reducing rehospitalization, with follow-up visits within 7 days or less of hospital discharge, cited for example, as a quality measure for the American Heart Association's "Get with the Guidelines, Target: Heart Failure" initiative.[20] Yet organizations struggle to implement this seemingly straightforward process for patients across the board. Part of Northwestern Medicine's multidisciplinary heart failure transition team intervention included ensuring that all patients identified in the at-risk population had improved post-discharge ambulatory follow-up based on individual need. Queuing theory was used to analyze hospital discharge load, and understand the capacity needed in clinic to reduce wait times and improve access for the cardiology clinic. Modest "buffering" of clinic capacity led to significant increases in patients scheduled within 7 and 14 days of discharge.[21]

WHAT'S NEXT?

Although the pace of change is perhaps not as rapid as some had expected, the federal government continues to pursue an aggressive agenda to expand a portfolio of both voluntary and mandatory government-based APMs. Commercial payers, and increasingly large employers, continue to follow suit. Whether in the population-based "accountable care" domain or in the episode-based "bundled care" domain, the basic premise is to migrate the health care delivery system, using financial incentives for improved outcomes. The real challenge is accelerating and scaling micro-care delivery redesign and process improvements at a macro level. Beyond understanding the data and the sources of clinical variation, systems-level financial investment, operational commitment, and an overarching will to change the status quo are required.

Creating and implementing models of care across episodes that achieve the Quadruple Aim remains a work-in-progress, but if done well, it can augment the biomedical innovation and discoveries that advance our understanding of the pathophysiology of a complex disease like heart failure.

DISCLOSURE

The authors have nothing to disclose.

REFERENCES

1. MITRE Corporation. Health care payment learning & action network. 2019. Available at: https://hcp-lan.org/workproducts/apm-methodology-2019.pdf. Accessed February, 2020.
2. Centers for Medicare & Medicaid Services. Inpatient Prospective Payment System (IPPS) Provider Summary for All Diagnosis-Related Groups (DRG) - FY2017. Baltimore, MD. 2019. Available at: https://data.cms.gov/Medicare-Inpatient/Inpatient-Prospective-Payment-System-IPPS-Provider/tcsp-6e99. Accessed February, 2020.
3. Centers for Medicare and Medicaid Services. National Health Expenditure Data. NHE Summary, including share of GDP, CY 1960-2018. 2019. Available at: https://www.cms.gov/Research-Statistics-Data-and-Systems/Statistics-Trends-and-Reports/NationalHealthExpendData/NationalHealthAccountsHistorical. Accessed February, 2020.
4. Sawyer B, Cox C. How does health spending in the U.S. compare to other countries? Peterson-KFF Health System Tracker. 2018. Available at: https://www.healthsystemtracker.org/chart-collection/health-spending-u-s-compare-countries/#item-u-s-increased-public-private-sector-spending-faster-rate-similar-countries. Accessed February, 2020.
5. Papanicolas I, Woskie LR, Jha AK. March). Health care spending in the United States and other high-income countries. JAMA 2018;319(10):1024–39.
6. Anderson GF, Reinhardt UE, Hussey PS, et al. It's the prices, stupid: why the United States is so different

from other countries. Health Aff 2003;22(3). https://doi.org/10.1377/hlthaff.22.3.89.

7. Skinner JS, Gottlieb DJ, Carmichael D. A New Series of Medicare Expenditure Measures by Hospital Referral Region: 2003-2008. The Dartmouth Atlast Project. (K. K. Bronner, Ed.) Hanover, NH. 2011. Available at: https://www.dartmouthatlas.org/downloads/reports/PA_Spending_Report_0611.pdf. Accessed February, 2020.

8. Goodman DC, Fisher ES, Chiang-Hu C. After hospitalization: a Dartmouth Atlas Report on post-acute care for medicare beneficiaries. The Darmouth Atlas. (K. K. Bronner, Ed.) Hanover, NH. 2011. Available at: https://www.dartmouthatlas.org/downloads/reports/Post_discharge_events_092811.pdf. Accessed February, 2020.

9. Chen LM, Norton EC, Banerjee M, et al. Surgical post-acute care spending driven by choice of post-acute care setting rather than intensity of services. Health Aff 2017;36(1):83–90.

10. Office of Inspector General. Medicare Hospital Prospective Payment System: How DRG Rates Are Calculated and Updated . (P. Gottlober, Ed.). 2001. Available at: https://oig.hhs.gov/oei/reports/oei-09-00-00200.pdf. Accessed February, 2020.

11. Centers for Medicare & Medicaid Services. Acute care episode demonstration. P.L. 108-173. Baltimore, MD. 2008. Available at: https://innovation.cms.gov/Files/x/ACE-Solicitation.pdf. Accessed February, 2020.

12. Patient Protection and Affordable Care Act. (2010). 42 U.S.C. § 18001.

13. McCarthy M. Obama administration sets goals for Medicare's shift to "value based" payment. BMJ 2015;350. https://doi.org/10.1136/bmj.h486.

14. Bodenheimer T, Sinsky C. From triple to quadruple aim: care of the patient requires care of the provider. Ann Fam Med 2014;12(6):573–6.

15. Benjamin EJ, Muntner P, Alonso A, et al. Heart disease and stroke statistics—2019 update: a report from the American Heart Association. Circulation 2019;139(10):e56–538.

16. Centers for Disease Control and Prevention. Heart Disease. 2019. Heart Disease Resources for Health Professionals: Available at: https://www.cdc.gov/heartdisease/heart_failure.htm. Accessed February, 2020.

17. Ahmad FS, Wehbe RM, Kansal P, et al. Targeting the correct population when designing transitional care programs for Medicare patients hospitalized with heart failure. JAMA Cardiol 2017;2(11):1274–5.

18. Mutharasan R, Kansal P, Benacka C, et al. Abstract 152: enterprise data warehouse-supported early identification of acute decompensated heart failure admissions for efficient and multidisciplinary transitional care team interventions. Circ Cardiovasc Qual Outcomes 2016;9(Suppl_2):A152.

19. Fine M, Mutharasan R, Kansal P, et al. Pharmacist-led transition of care interventions identify and reduce medication errors in heart failure patients post-discharge. J Card Fail 2016;22(8):S134–5.

20. American Heart Association. Get with the Guidelines: Heart Failure. 2018. Available at: https://www.heart.org/-/media/files/professional/quality-improvement/get-with-the-guidelines/get-with-the-guidelines-hf/educational-materials/hf-fact-sheet_updated-011119_v2.pdf?la=en&hash=1E39EB095FD5A513D1C3D19B22B48CEE3C6AF4B9. Accessed February, 2020.

21. Mutharasan R, Ahmad FS, Gurvich I, et al. Buffer or suffer: redesigning heart failure postdischarge clinic using queuing theory. Circ Cardiovasc Qual Outcomes 2018;11(7):e004351.

Statement of Ownership, Management, and Circulation
UNITED STATES POSTAL SERVICE® (All Periodicals Publications Except Requester Publications)

1. Publication Title	2. Publication Number	3. Filing Date
HEART FAILURE CLINICS	025 – 055	9/18/2020

4. Issue Frequency	5. Number of Issues Published Annually	6. Annual Subscription Price
JAN, APR, JUL, OCT	4	$269.00

7. Complete Mailing Address of Known Office of Publication (Not printer) (Street, city, county, state, and ZIP+4®)

ELSEVIER INC.
230 Park Avenue, Suite 800
New York, NY 10169

Contact Person: Malathi Samayan
Telephone (Include area code): 91-44-4299-4507

8. Complete Mailing Address of Headquarters or General Business Office of Publisher (Not printer)

ELSEVIER INC.
230 Park Avenue, Suite 800
New York, NY 10169

9. Full Names and Complete Mailing Addresses of Publisher, Editor, and Managing Editor (Do not leave blank)

Publisher (Name and complete mailing address)

DOLORES MELONI ELSEVIER INC.
1600 JOHN F KENNEDY BLVD. SUITE 1800
PHILADELPHIA, PA 19103-2899

Editor (Name and complete mailing address)

JOANNA COLLETT, ELSEVIER INC.
1600 JOHN F KENNEDY BLVD. SUITE 1800
PHILADELPHIA, PA 19103-2899

Managing Editor (Name and complete mailing address)

PATRICK MANLEY, ELSEVIER INC.
1600 JOHN F KENNEDY BLVD. SUITE 1800
PHILADELPHIA, PA 19103-2899

10. Owner (Do not leave blank. If the publication is owned by a corporation, give the name and address of the corporation immediately followed by the names and addresses of all stockholders owning or holding 1 percent or more of the total amount of stock. If not owned by a corporation, give the names and addresses of the individual owners. If owned by a partnership or other unincorporated firm, give its name and address as well as those of each individual owner. If the publication is published by a nonprofit organization, give its name and address.)

Full Name	Complete Mailing Address
WHOLLY OWNED SUBSIDIARY OF REED/ELSEVIER, US HOLDINGS	1600 JOHN F KENNEDY BLVD. SUITE 1800 PHILADELPHIA, PA 19103-2899

11. Known Bondholders, Mortgagees, and Other Security Holders Owning or Holding 1 Percent or More of Total Amount of Bonds, Mortgages, or Other Securities. If none, check box ► ☐ None

Full Name	Complete Mailing Address
N/A	

12. Tax Status (For completion by nonprofit organizations authorized to mail at nonprofit rates) (Check one)
The purpose, function, and nonprofit status of this organization and the exempt status for federal income tax purposes:
☒ Has Not Changed During Preceding 12 Months
☐ Has Changed During Preceding 12 Months (Publisher must submit explanation of change with this statement)

PS Form 3526, July 2014 (Page 1 of 4 (see instructions page 4)) PSN 7530-01-000-9931 PRIVACY NOTICE: See our privacy policy on www.usps.com

---

13. Publication Title	14. Issue Date for Circulation Data Below
HEART FAILURE CLINICS	JULY 2020

15. Extent and Nature of Circulation			Average No. Copies Each Issue During Preceding 12 Months	No. Copies of Single Issue Published Nearest to Filing Date
a. Total Number of Copies (Net press run)			36	31
b. Paid Circulation (By Mail and Outside the Mail)	(1)	Mailed Outside-County Paid Subscriptions Stated on PS Form 3541 (Include paid distribution above nominal rate, advertiser's proof copies, and exchange copies)	18	16
	(2)	Mailed In-County Paid Subscriptions Stated on PS Form 3541 (Include paid distribution above nominal rate, advertiser's proof copies, and exchange copies)	0	0
	(3)	Paid Distribution Outside the Mails Including Sales Through Dealers and Carriers, Street Vendors, Counter Sales, and Other Paid Distribution Outside USPS®	10	9
	(4)	Paid Distribution by Other Classes of Mail Through the USPS (e.g. First-Class Mail®)	0	0
c. Total Paid Distribution (Sum of 15b (1), (2), (3), and (4))		►	28	25
d. Free or Nominal Rate Distribution (By Mail and Outside the Mail)	(1)	Free or Nominal Rate Outside-County Copies included on PS Form 3541	8	6
	(2)	Free or Nominal Rate In-County Copies Included on PS Form 3541	0	0
	(3)	Free or Nominal Rate Copies Mailed at Other Classes Through the USPS (e.g. First-Class Mail)	0	0
	(4)	Free or Nominal Rate Distribution Outside the Mail (Carriers or other means)	0	0
e. Total Free or Nominal Rate Distribution (Sum of 15d (1), (2), (3) and (4))		►	8	6
f. Total Distribution (Sum of 15c and 15e)		►	36	31
g. Copies not Distributed (See Instructions to Publishers #4 (page #3))		►	0	0
h. Total (Sum of 15f and g)		►	36	31
i. Percent Paid (15c divided by 15f times 100)		►	77.77%	80.64%

* If you are claiming electronic copies, go to line 16 on page 3. If you are not claiming electronic copies, skip to line 17 on page 3.

16. Electronic Copy Circulation	Average No. Copies Each Issue During Preceding 12 Months	No. Copies of Single Issue Published Nearest to Filing Date
a. Paid Electronic Copies	►	
b. Total Paid Print Copies (Line 15c) + Paid Electronic Copies (Line 16a)	►	
c. Total Print Distribution (Line 15f) + Paid Electronic Copies (Line 16a)	►	
d. Percent Paid (Both Print & Electronic Copies) (16b divided by 16c × 100)	►	

☒ I certify that 50% of all my distributed copies (electronic and print) are paid above a nominal price.

17. Publication of Statement of Ownership
☒ If the publication is a general publication, publication of this statement is required. Will be printed in the OCTOBER 2020 issue of this publication. ☐ Publication not required.

18. Signature and Title of Editor, Publisher, Business Manager, or Owner

Malathi Samayan - Distribution Controller

Malathi Samayan   Date 9/18/2020

I certify that all information furnished on this form is true and complete. I understand that anyone who furnishes false or misleading information on this form or who omits material or information requested on the form may be subject to criminal sanctions (including fines and imprisonment) and/or civil sanctions (including civil penalties).

PS Form 3526, July 2014 (Page 3 of 4) PRIVACY NOTICE: See our privacy policy on www.usps.com

Printed and bound by CPI Group (UK) Ltd, Croydon, CR0 4YY

03/10/2024

01040306-0009